CRUNCH

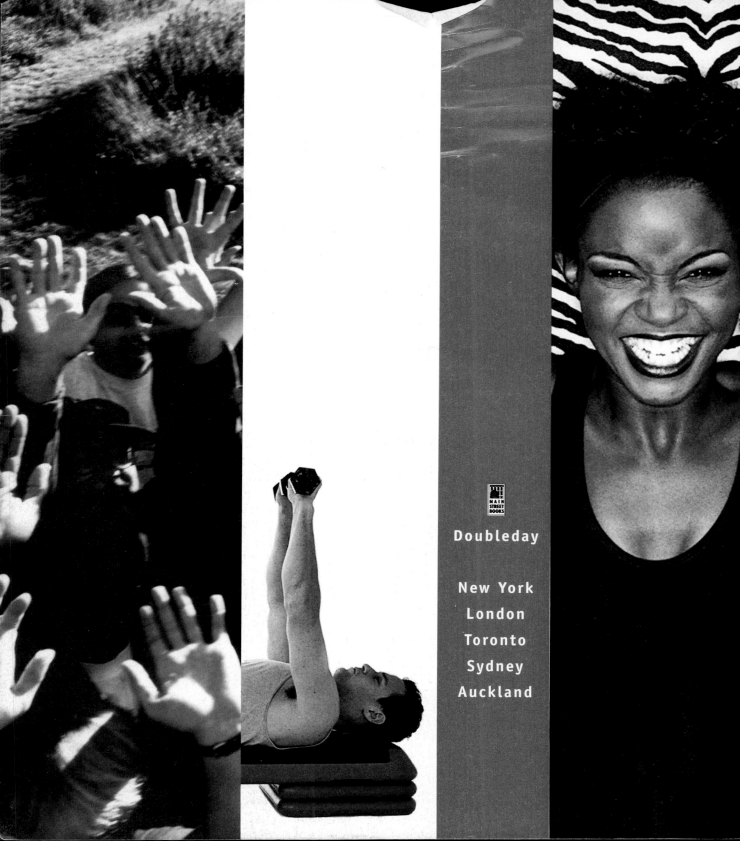

MAIN
STREET
BOOKS

Doubleday

New York
London
Toronto
Sydney
Auckland

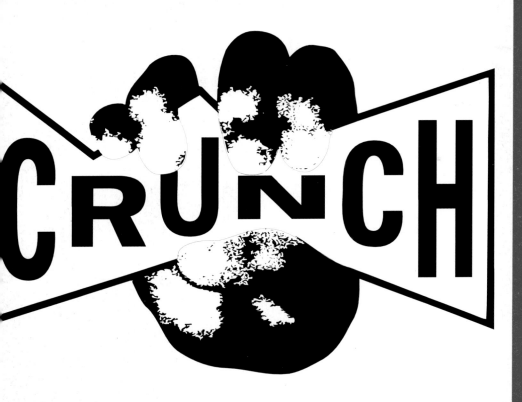

CRUNCH

Liz

Neporent

with

John

Egan

A Complete Guide to Health and Fitness

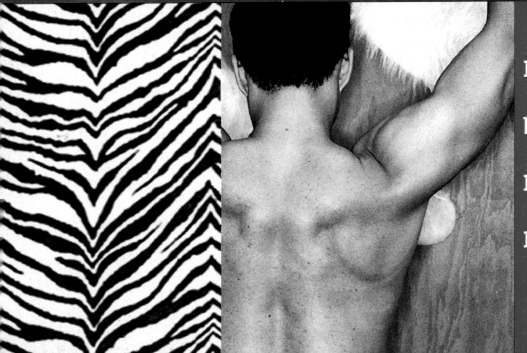

Photographs

by

Daniel

Kron

A Main Street Book

Published by Doubleday

a division of Bantam Doubleday Dell Publishing Group, Inc.

1540 Broadway, New York, New York 10036

Main Street Books, **Doubleday**, and the portrayal of a building with a tree are trademarks of Doubleday, a division of Bantam Doubleday Dell Publishing Group, Inc.

Book design by Amanda Kavanagh

Library of Congress Cataloging-in-Publication Data

Neporent, Liz.

   Crunch: a complete guide to health and fitness / Liz Neporent with John Egan. — 1st ed.

        p.   cm.

   "A Main Street book"—T.p. verso.

   1. Physical fitness.   2. Health.   3. Aerobic exercises.
4. Nutrition.   I. Egan, John, 1965–   .   II. Title.

GV481.N397   1997

613.7—dc20   96-30821

                              CIP1

ISBN 0-385-48809-2

Printed in the United States of America

February 1997

10 9 8 7 6 5 4 3 2 1

First Edition

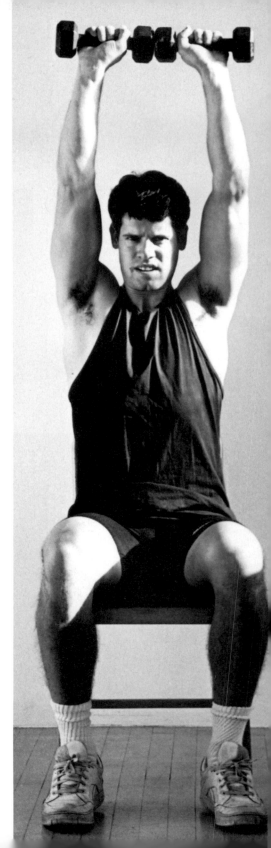

From Liz Neporent

Many thanks to my Frontline Fitness coworkers Holly Byrne, Bob Welter, and Nancy Ngui for picking up the slack and spurring me on during the writing of this and previous books. My terrific parents, mother-in-law, and various brothers and sisters have also been extremely encouraging, as have my good friends Richard and Amy Miller from the Gym Source in New York City.

To Doug Levine: I appreciate the opportunity to work on this book and with the Crunch organization. To Sarah Dent: You are the most organized, efficient person I've ever met—thanks for everything; you can go home now. To the models who dragged their butts downtown to be photographed: You all look great! Make sure you thank Dan Kron, our phenomenal photographer, for that.

Finally, to my husband, Jay Shafran: You're the best. Thanks for helping out with everything and anything, but most of all, thanks for walking the dog.

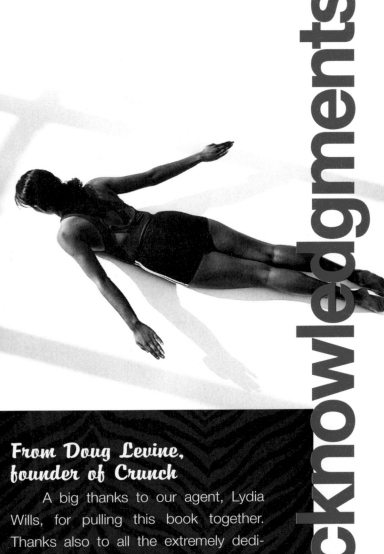

From Doug Levine, founder of Crunch

A big thanks to our agent, Lydia Wills, for pulling this book together. Thanks also to all the extremely dedicated and diligent staff at Crunch. Running Crunch is a little like putting on a Broadway show, and the hard work of the staff, including the gym maintenance staff, sales team, front desk staff, managers, instructors, and all the staff in the Corporate office, ensures that the curtain goes up on time and that we play to a full house every day. Cheers!

acknowledgments

contents

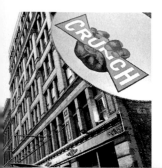

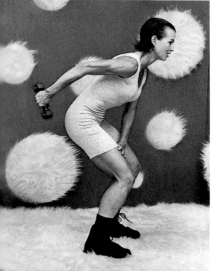
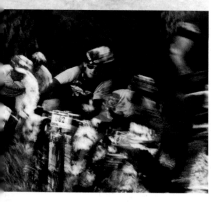

contents

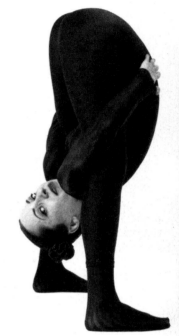

strength training for weight control and toning

Learn how lifting weights and using resistance bands and a step bench increase your strength, build lean muscle mass, control your weight, and sculpt your body. Pick a routine that suits your lifestyle. Note that this chapter does not include abdominal exercises—those you'll learn in the next chapter.

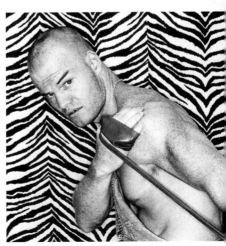

contents

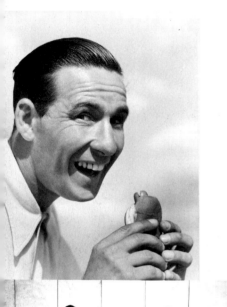

contents

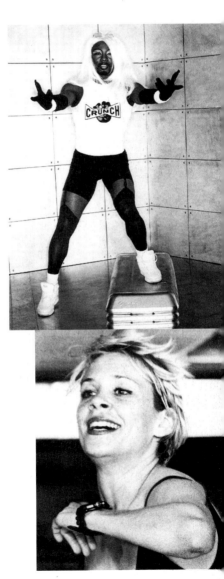

107 4 guts!
how to define and tone your abdominal muscles

Abs are such a large, complex muscle group that they need their own chapter. Learn how abs work together and support your spine. Learn how to safely condition and define with special, concentrated exercises.

contents

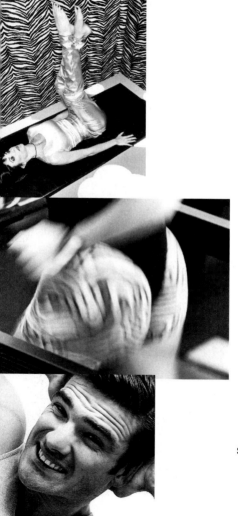

5 spine! 127

strengthening your spine for good posture and well-being

Learn how good posture makes you more fit and improves your self-image. Find out how the spine shrinks and combat this with exercise.

contents

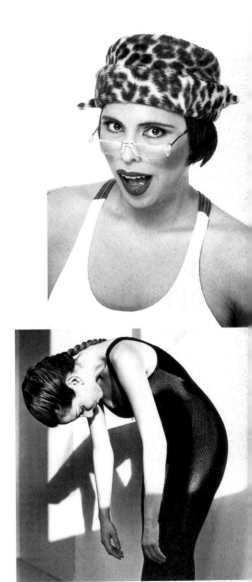

contents

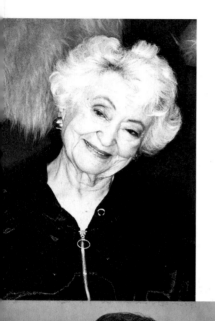

Hamstring Stretch: *great for backs of thighs! makes your back feel better!*
Hip Roll: *loosens up the entire spine plus your hips, butt, and outer thighs!*
Back Release: *perfect for releasing tension all along your spine!*
Cobra: *stretches your abdominals and the tops of your thighs!*
Half a Hug: *stretches your upper back, shoulders, and the fronts of your upper arms!*
Forward Reach: *stretches your arm, wrist, and fingers!*
The Warrior: *a super-duper stretch for your whole upper body and lower back!*
Side Stretch: *stretches out your obliques, your spine, and your upper back!*
Quad Stretch: *good for stretching your thighs and hips!*
Wall Press: *sheer heaven for your ankles and calves!*

7 chow! 163
a lesson in nutrition, fat, and calorie intake

Learn how a healthy diet makes you fit faster and how to incorporate one into your lifestyle. Learn about calorie intake, protein, carbs, fats, cholesterol, sodium, plus little-known weight-loss tips. Learn how to combine all this into a healthy, real-life, everyday eating program.

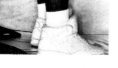

contents

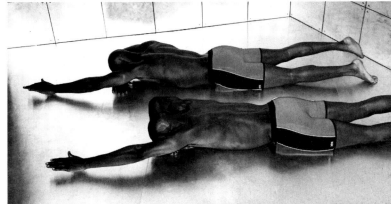

huh?

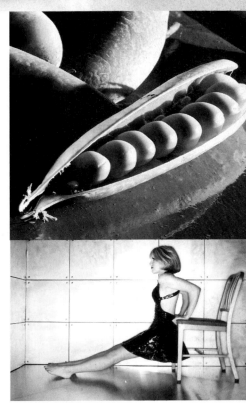

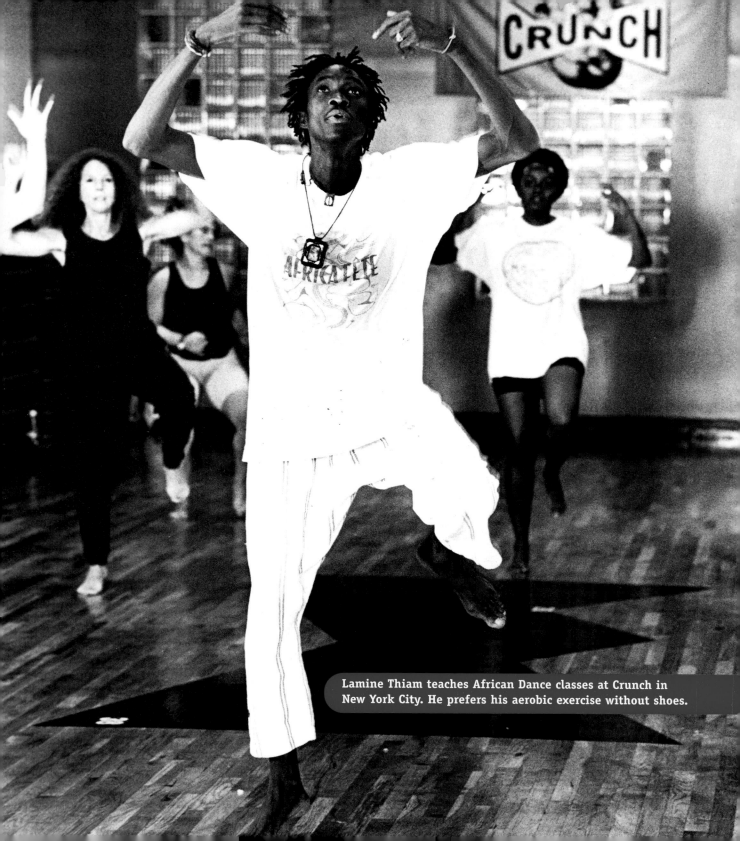

Lamine Thiam teaches African Dance classes at Crunch in New York City. He prefers his aerobic exercise without shoes.

Crunch!
It's a Movement!

Crunch is a gym in New York—not one of those cruisers and bruisers gyms, but a user-friendly, home-away-from-home kind of gym. More than that, Crunch now represents a whole new approach to fitness, one that's helped energize and transform the way hundreds of people exercise.

The idea for Crunch is simple: Everyone Is Welcome. We don't care who you are, and we don't care what you look like. We don't care what kind of job you have, or where you live, or whom you're sleeping with. We're not here to tell you you're not cool enough, or pretty enough, or rich enough. If you're motivated, we'll help you get in shape. If not, we may even help you get motivated, but we're not going to be bullies about it. Don't let the name mislead you: Crunch is not one of those sadistic spandex regimes. All we want is to get you moving, get your heart beating and your lungs pumping, your muscles working and your mind stretching.

Our slogan is *Crunch: It's a Movement.* See, it's a double entendre: a movement like an exercise and a movement like people coming together and experiencing a change of consciousness . . . oh, you know what we mean. The point is that Crunch is about more than just gym stuff. We believe if you have a chance to exercise, you end up healthier, and happier, and with a better body to boot.

So you say you're not built like Cindy Crawford. Don't worry. Few of us are. When most of us look in the mirror, we see a distortion based on our doubts and based on society's notion of the beautiful body that we couldn't possibly live up to.

In fact, we're all very different. Some of us are clumsy and some are lazy; some of us smoke too much, and some of us sleep too little; and some of us have skinny little arms, some of us have big asses. Okay. But you can still be the healthiest, strongest, happiest, clumsy-

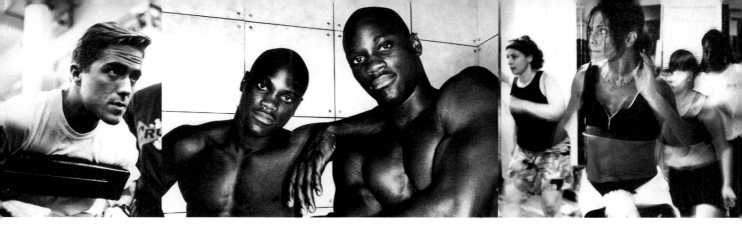

lazy-tired-skinny-armed-big-assed person you can be.

What's more, we all have different desires, expectations, abilities, and tolerances. And since fitness should be a lifelong activity, why spend your life doing someone else's workout? It's your body, and we believe in helping you find the program that's right for it—your exercises, your diet, at your speed. That's what this book is for. Think of it as a guide to making the best of yourself.

Most important, we think exercise should be fun. Believe it or not, the time you spend training can be enjoyable, engaging, even interesting. To prove it, we've put together a set of routines that ought to keep you entertained. That way, you can exercise not just your muscles but your mind, your personality, your spirit, because you can have all the muscles in the world and still be out of shape if you don't feel beautiful and confident. You know all those ridiculous New Age platitudes about looking good and feeling good, being spiritually tuned up and in harmony with the universe? We know they're ridiculous. We know they're platitudes. But we believe them anyway.

Seven years ago, we opened a tiny fitness studio in Manhattan's East Village, just a funky little spot with a few new ideas: that exercise could be more than just the same old sweaty grind and that fitness could be more than just bulging biceps and flat bellies. With the help of a lot of creative instructors, we offered classes in everything from gospel aerobics to specific sport training to yoga cycling. Our teachers were not only experts but rappers, modern dancers, and professional boxers.

And people came. Men and women,

Marc Goodman teaches a class called Cuttin' Up. He says, "I try to make aerobics more fun for my students with my good looks, remarkable wit, gut-splitting jokes. Like that last joke, for example."

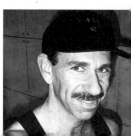

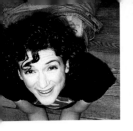

Terry Walsh taught Diva Step aerobics at Crunch in New York. Says Terry, "Crunch is different because we're encouraged to make our classes entertaining. No idea is too weird, as long as it helps people get fit."

young and old, thin people and not thin people. We attracted Hasidim, Hell's Angels, pimply kids, housewives, supermodels, and store clerks. Boho types too: artists, musicians, dancers, and designers. Deborah Harry came; so did Betsey Johnson. And yeah, so did Cindy Crawford.

Soon we expanded into five big gyms in New York, one in Los Angeles, and we now have thousands of happy members. And even though what you're holding isn't a gym, that's okay, because you don't need a gym to use this book. It's designed to be used at home. (It's all part of our plan to take over the world; one body at a time.)

A lot of people worked together to bring you this book. Liz Neporent wrote and put together the exercises: she's a renowned, certified fitness consultant with a master's degree in exercise physiology, the author of an award-winning and best-selling fitness guide called *Buns of Steel* as well as *Shape* magazine's *Do It Right!* video series, and a frequent contributor to a number of health and fitness magazines. And then there are all the instructors, members, and assorted free spirits, savants, and visionaries who've helped us develop the program from the beginning. Since they'll be the ones who'll be explaining the Crunch way of life, you'll meet them individually on the following pages. When you get down to it, that's what we hope this book will bring you; a way of life. So go ahead and jump in. What the hell, have a ball.

Doug Levine

—Doug Levine, founder of Crunch

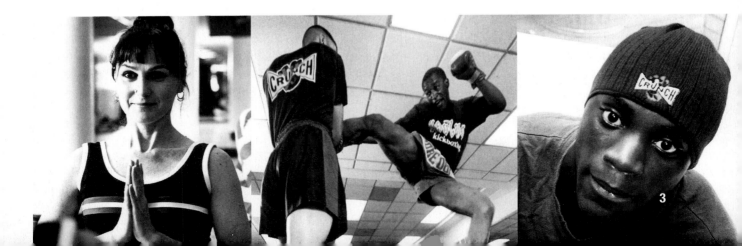

3

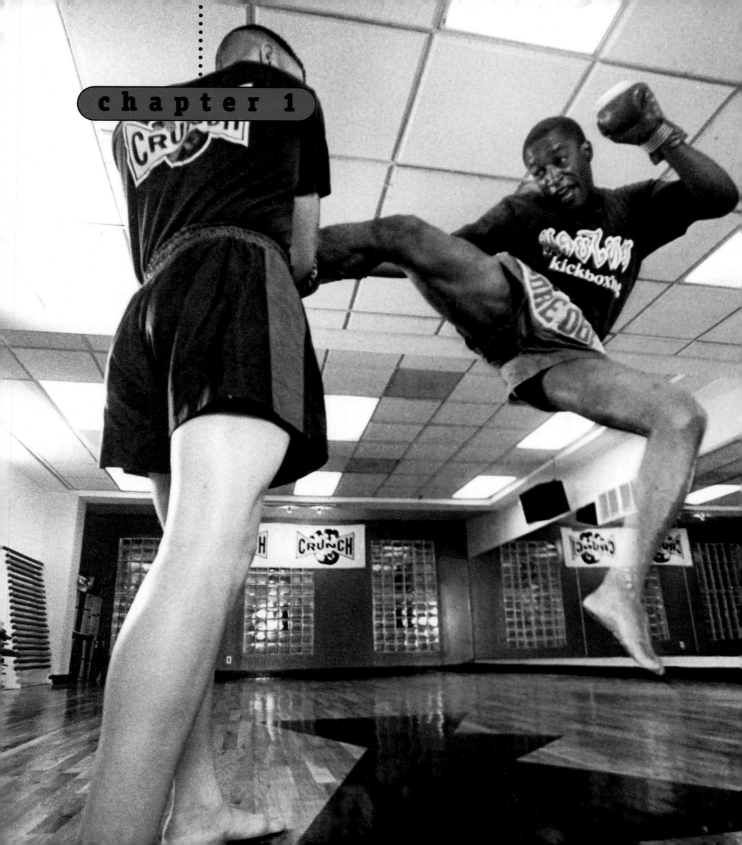

flesh!

Determining Your Body Shape and a Plan for Reshaping It

Genetics, Fat, and Greener Pastures

Two 5'4" women, both weighing 135 pounds, stand next to you in one of those weird open dressing rooms. One wears a size 6, one a size 10. Why? Well, the scale gives you only a partial snapshot of your body composition. How much fat vs. how much lean body tissue you possess is what determines the size and shape. Do you dream of being a size 6 and then find yourself envying the well-proportioned, voluptuous size 10? There's a big difference between the "Did you see me win the Pro Beach Volleyball Tournament?" size 10 and a "Is anyone going to eat these last seven doughnuts?" size 10. This is a result of whether you pack primarily fat or muscle into your dress size.

Your lean body tissue consists of bones, organs, and muscle tissue. Fat weight consists of the essential fat that pads and protects your organs and the excess body fat you store all over. While your fat distribution is partially dictated by genetics, it's also influenced over a lifetime by diet, exercise, and lifestyle habits (do you take the elevator up two flights to get to the StairMaster?).

Also, in addition to genetics and diet, there's the natural aging process. Now, just in case the clock isn't already ticking loud enough, listen to this. Beginning in our mid-twenties we lose half a pound of muscle and gain a pound of fat each year, a net weight gain of *five pounds per decade.* (Does that mean you gain twenty pounds listening to your soft and easy favorites from the sixties, seventies, eighties, and nineties?) Lost muscle tissue does result in a *slower metabolism,* making perpetual weight gain virtually inevitable. Before you lose the will to work out, however, there are ways to combat Mother Nature's sick sense of humor.

The Shape You're Born With: Different Natural Body Types

The way humans are shaped falls into one of three broad categories: *endomorph, ectomorph,* or *mesomorph.* Scientists call this *somatotyping.* Understanding your somatotype will help you in training, as you'll know what type of results to expect. Most people are a combination of all three types, though you tend to resemble one the most. Your appearance will change as you lose fat and gain muscle, but your basic shape is determined by genetics.

Endomorph:

Endomorphs have round, smooth bodies and large bones. Their hips are wider than their shoulders and their weight is concentrated below the waist. When in shape, endomorphs look toned and muscular but not ripped. Endomorphs usually have a hard time striving for the lower ends of the body-fat spectrum. Sticking to a low-fat diet will help maintain weight. Strength training keeps the metabolic ball rolling and helps balance body proportions. High-calorie-burning aerobic sessions trim off body fat.

Ectomorph:

If you're an ectomorph, you're slender, with shoulders and hips that are approximately the same width. You have a small-to-medium frame and tend toward an angular look with some muscle definition but not a lot of size. Other types envy your ability to repel excess body fat, but your body may also resist the development of

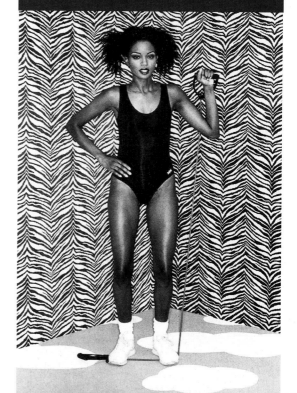

Tomiko, a successful fashion model, is a classic ectomorph. Many models are, due to their low body fat and naturally small, thin frame. Tomiko does some light aerobics to keep her lovely delicate body in shape. She feels lucky to be naturally thin, although she often wishes she was a bit more strong and muscular. You'll see her doing strength-training exercises in the next chapter to fill her out a bit.

lean muscle. You can probably take in more calories than other body types, but you should still watch dietary fat, cholesterol, and sodium for health reasons. You'll probably have to focus on weight training more than the other body types if you want to build strength and lean muscle tissue. Since weight loss isn't a problem, you probably don't need to spend hours and hours doing aerobics unless your goals are predominantly athletic.

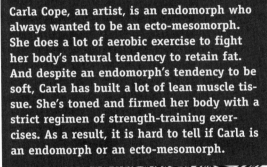

Mesomorph:

This is the most "athletic"-looking of the three types. He or she has a muscular, rectangular outline with strong bones and broad shoulders. Weight is distributed fairly evenly, with hips not quite

Luke MadDog Massey, a personal trainer, is a classic V-shaped, muscular mesomorph. As a trainer, he has further built his muscle mass and is in amazing shape. While he's satisfied with his body shape, sometimes he dreams of being a graceful endo-ectomorph ballerina. You'll see MadDog doing ab exercises and other strength-training exercises in the next chapter to tighten and tone his already tight and toned morph.

Carla Cope, an artist, is an endomorph who always wanted to be an ecto-mesomorph. She does a lot of aerobic exercise to fight her body's natural tendency to retain fat. And despite an endomorph's tendency to be soft, Carla has built a lot of lean muscle tissue. She's toned and firmed her body with a strict regimen of strength-training exercises. As a result, it is hard to tell if Carla is an endomorph or an ecto-mesomorph.

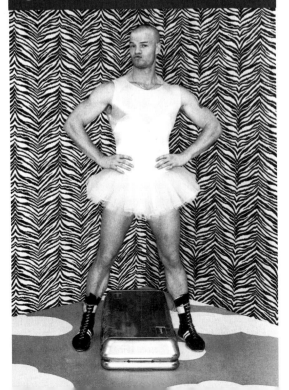

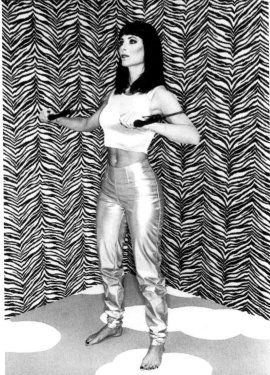

7

as wide as shoulders. Fit mesomorphs have size and definition. As a mesomorph, you can quickly fine-tune your body's athleticism. You can probably place equal emphasis on aerobics and strength work, but you'll have to watch the calorie and fat intake. Out-of-shape mesomorphs tend to look stocky.

Before you start somatotyping yourself based on your self-esteem, keep reading. Yes, you now understand the role body composition plays in how you look . . . but understand that body composition is only one component of being fit. There are five factors that affect your fitness level: body composition (as discussed), diet, aerobics, strength, and flexibility. The next section will discuss these factors so that you can use them to effectively transform that person you go to sleep with and wake up with every day of your life. After you learn about them, you'll take a test to assess your current fitness level and help you record the changes you make in the future.

The Five Fitness Factors

Doctors and other health specialists define fitness as your ability to function successfully in your given environment. Some peo-

ple translate that into a strict, holistic, organic, microbiotic, high-sweat, zero-fat approach to living. For others, fitness is cutting back to one pack a day. However, most experts agree on the *five fitness factors* which have the greatest influence on your ability to function physically. They're all equally important. To get 100 percent fit, you're going to have to clean out the attic of your mind so that all five can move in and live there.

Aerobic Conditioning

"Aerobic" is a term coined in the late sixties by an army doctor to refer to any sustained movement which relies on oxygen (air) for power—walking, running, skating, or swimming, for example. Consistent aerobic or cardiovascular exercise keeps your heart and lungs in good working order. It revs up your stamina. It helps lower your weight, your stress levels, your blood pressure, and your total cholesterol. It increases your energy level and decreases your need for sleep. It can improve your outlook and your self-esteem. (And if all that isn't enough, it puts your inner child in a really good mood.)

According to the American College of Sports Medicine (ACSM), to achieve a reasonably good level of aerobic fitness and gain immunity from heart disease and related illnesses, you need to do at least

8

three 20-minute sessions a week. You'll need to do more than that if you want to lose weight or run a marathon.

Strength

Strength isn't just overinflated oily guys in Speedos. Having a sufficient amount of strength is more practical than that. It's what enables you to gracefully hoist your overpacked carry-on into the overhead bin while thirty-five rows of businessmen watch you. Regular strength workouts pack lean muscle tissue onto your frame, which keeps your metabolism speedy as you get older and helps your body retain its tone and firmness. In the long run, strength training helps prevent osteoporosis by contributing to the preservation of bone density. To build strength, you must overload your muscles with some form of resistance or weight—like a dumbbell, barbell, exercise band, or weight machine. The ACSM recommends doing at least two strength-training sessions a week designed to stress all your major muscle groups, including your buttocks, thighs, lower legs, abdominals, lower back, chest, shoulders, and arms. Be prepared to spend a lot more time pumping iron than that if you're interested in body-building or power lifting.

Flexibility

Your flexibility means how tight or loose you are—the distance you can comfortably move your joints and muscles. This depends on several things: your age, your activity level, and the structure of your joints. Improving or maintaining flexibility takes regular sessions of slow, static stretching. While it's never been proven that good flexibility prevents injury and muscle soreness, limbering up often reduces or prevents lower-back pain. Besides, many people find stretching relaxing in and of itself. Most experts, top athletes, and dancers recommend stretching for at least 5–10 minutes daily, at the end of a workout when your muscles are the warmest and most pliable.

Nutrition

Eating right is more than reduction, limitation, sacrifice, and avoidance. (Don't think "dieting.") You can get all the essential nutrients you need to fuel your body in tasty, enjoyable meals. (Think "balancing.") Don't count calories and fat grams. Cultivate good eating habits. Proper nutrition gives you more energy, prevents you from getting sick, and provides the building blocks for constructing a fit, healthy body. Cultivate a different attitude about eating. Next time you start to chow down, think about parts of your body. Think about your hungry heart, your needy muscles, your thirsty cells, your famished skin, and the other parts of you that hope you'll feed them with kindness and care. Eating badly doesn't just make being naked in front of people less fun. It also hurts the parts of you that you need to keep going and keep you healthy and happy for the rest of your life.

Body Composition

The closest you can come to accurately measuring your body fat is with a method called "hydrostatic weighing." This involves getting dunked in a tub to see how much water you displace. (Fat floats; muscle sinks and therefore displaces more water.) If outfitting your home with a dunking booth from the state fair is inconvenient or impractical, the next-best thing is having various areas of your body pinched with an instrument called a "caliper." Even if you're able to find a friend willing to pinch your fat, chances are the temptation to pretend they're an angry, vengeful lobster or an enormous crab will prove too much. Fat pinching should be done by an experienced professional who will add up the thicknesses of the fat pinched and calculate the results using a formula. Skilled body-fat takers can be found in cutting-edge health clubs and hospital weight-loss programs. You can roughly estimate your own body-fat percentage with the simple test in the next section. It's not as accurate as caliper measuring but it's a good way of keeping track of improvement as you become more fit.

Factor this: Dancers who can't lift a heavy box aren't fit. Bodybuilders who can't run around the block aren't fit. A fitness program should not focus on only one fitness factor. Not all fitness factors require equal time—just the *right* amount of time. What's the right amount of time? Depends on what you need to work on.

Pre-Fitness Test Pep Talk

Take the simple tests on the next few pages. It'll take you about half an hour. You'll need a pencil, our Comparison Box, a watch with a second hand, a tape measure, and some masking tape. Avoid physical activity, smoking, caffeine, and alcohol for up to four hours before you take the tests. Once you've been working out for a while, redo the evaluation and compare the results. Results vary depending upon how much exercise time you've put in and what you've been eating—but you should see improvements. Pay attention to the areas that didn't improve so much; you'll get an idea of which factors need more attention. Most people see noticeable results in all factors the first six weeks of working out and making lifestyle changes, so take your second test in six weeks and then every three months thereafter.

fitness test

Note: This self-evaluation is t give you a ballpark idea of you fitness level. It is not a substitut for medical tests by your docto If you haven't exercised in a whil or have a history of health prob lems, check with your doctor be fore taking this test or beginnin an exercise program.

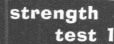

strength
test 1

Push-ups
(Upper-Body Strength)

Men, do as many full push-ups as you can without stopping or pausing; women, do as many knee push-ups as you can without stopping or pausing. Record the amount in the Comparison Box.

How to do full push-ups: Lie on your stomach with your palms on the floor, directly in front of your shoulders. Then push your entire body up off the floor so you're balanced on your palms and toes. Remember to pull your abdominal muscles in slightly and keep your back flat. Lower to begin.

How to do knee push-ups: Lie on your stomach with your lower legs off the floor, ankles crossed. Push your entire body off the floor so you're balanced on your palms and knees. Lower to begin. Record the number you can do in the Comparison Box.

strength
test 2

Crunches (Abdominal and Lower-Back Strength)

Lie on your back with your arms straight along your sides. Curl your head, neck, and shoulders up off the floor as you slide your hands forward along the floor. Record the number of repetitions you complete without stopping or pausing (or if you can't curl up all the way any longer) in the Comparison Box. If this test hurts your back, skip it.

erobic
conditioning

Mile Endurance Test

up by walking at an pace for a minute or so. the start of a measured ile course and set your atch at zero. Start your and begin walking or g or jogging as fast as an. Give your best effort you feel weak, sick, or stop! As you complete iles, stop your watch and down your time to the st second in the Com- on Box on page 14. If 1.5 seems like an unbeliev- far distance, choose thing shorter. The actual ce doesn't matter. You want a benchmark to improvement.

flexibility test

Sit and Reach Test (for Leg and Lower Back Flexibility)

Place a 12-inch piece of masking tape on the floor. Lay the tape measure so that it's perpendicular to the tape and so that it crosses the masking tape at the tape measure's 15-inch mark. Sit down with your legs straight, so that your feet are at opposite ends of the tape. Place one hand on top of the other, take a deep breath, exhale, and then stretch forward as far as you comfortably can. Make note of how far you move forward on the tape measure. Repeat three times and record your best score in the Comparison Box.

Height/Hip Method

Measure your height in inches to the nearest inch. Mark it on the "height" line in the chart below. Measure your hips around the widest girth to the nearest inch. Mark it on the "hip girth" line. With a ruler, draw a diagonal line from your height mark to your hip girth mark. Your body-fat percentage is indicated where your line crosses the "percent fat" column. Record this in the Comparison Box.

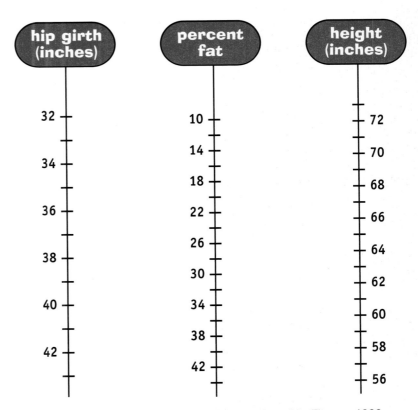

Reprinted by permission from J. H. Wilmore, *Sensible Fitness*, 1986 (Champaign, IL Human Kinetics Publishers), 31.

13

test	your score 1	your score 2	optimal score
Aerobic Conditioning			18 minutes or faster
Push-ups			23 or more repetitions
Crunches			40 or more repetitions
Sit and Reach			19 inches or more
Body-Fat Percentage			Men: 12%–20% Women: 16%–20%

Body-Type Test
Which Kind of Morph Are You?

1 Encircle your wrist using your middle finger and thumb. They:

  a. don't touch

  b. just touch

  c. touch with some overlapping

  d. wrap around twice (those are some mighty big fingers or you're missing a wrist)

2 Bend your elbow and make a muscle by tightening your fist. With your other hand, find the bulge of your upper arm that begins near the crease above your elbow. Using the width of your fingers, measure the distance between the start of this bulge and the crease in your arm. The distance is:

  a. one finger width

  b. two finger widths

  c. three finger widths or more

3 Stand sideways next to a mirror. Balance yourself on one leg standing as much on tiptoe as you can without falling over. Note the point at which the bulge of your calf muscle stops closest to your heel. Come down off tiptoe and look at where this point is in relation to the distance between the back of your heel and the back of your knee. Your calf muscle covers:

a. 3/4 the distance between the back of the knee and the heel

b. 1/2 the distance between the back of the knee and the heel

c. 1/4 the distance between the back of the knee and the heel

4 Measure your hips and waist. Subtract your waist from your hip measurement and do so without any frowning or grimacing. The difference is:

a. less than 2 inches

b. more than 2 but less than 8 inches

c. 8 inches or more

d. 3 yards or more (oh, my, that's going to take a little extra work)

5 With your arm hanging at your side, measure the largest part of your upper arm. Flex your arm (as you did in question 1) and measure at the same point. Subtract the hanging measurement from the flexed measurement. The difference between them is:

a. less than 1/4 inch

b. between 1/4 inch and 1 inch

c. more than 1 inch

6 Stand in front of a mirror and assess your body. It is:

a. rounded, especially around the hips, elbows, and knees. Your hips are wider than your shoulders. Most of your weight is concentrated in your hips and thighs.

b. has a muscular "rectangular" outline. Your shoulders are wider than your hips. Your weight is distributed more or less evenly between the upper and lower body.

c. sharp and angular, especially the elbows, hips, and knees. Your shoulders and hips are approximately the same width.

7 You are:

a. overweight

b. average weight

c. below average weight

Which morph are you? If you have three or more (a) answers, your body type is closest to endomorph. If you chose three or more (b) answers, your body is closest to mesomorph. If you chose three or more (c) answers, your body is closest to ectomorph. If your answers were more or less evenly spread between two types, consider yourself a true combination type, such as a meso-endomorph. Now that you have a silly word to describe your body, all that's left is to transform yours into the sexiest body possible for your particular morph.

A Sort-of Test: A Food Diary

Testing your nutrition factor is a little different than the fitness tests you just took. You won't need a pencil, our Comparison Box, a watch with a second hand, a tape measure, masking tape, or a tape of your favorite songs. Just try to be (somewhat) honest. While the best way to assess your eating habits is by visiting a registered dietitian, you can get a rough idea of your nutrition level by keeping a food diary. Write down everything you eat for three days, including at least one weekend day. Include portion size and all details. Don't just write "Salad." Write down "Large salad with croutons, lettuce, tomato, cheese, ham, and approximately 6 tablespoons of French dressing."

At the end of the three days, look over your intake. Although you might not be able to determine your exact calorie count or how much fat you've eaten, a sentimental journey of all the crap you put in your mouth in the last 72 hours (a trip down calorie lane) can be very eye-opening. Sometimes the simple act of writing

things down is enough to keep you eating right. You might want to consider keeping a long-term food diary.

Make a New Plan

Most of us jump into fitness programs with little notion of what we're trying to accomplish. Vague statements like "I want to lose weight" aren't real goals. Experts will tell you that lack of planning and unrealistic goals explain why more than 60 percent of people who begin an exercise program drop out within the first month and two out of three people who join a health club never go more than twice. It may also be part of the reason why 95 percent of diets fail.

Setting realistic goals and going after them is the number one way to stay motivated about your fitness program. "I want to attract a girlfriend" is not a goal that will make you stick to your program. Especially if you attract one. You know the old "I have a girlfriend now, so I don't have to worry about being a babe magnet anymore. Bring on the french fries! She loves me just the way I am."

You now have the tools to set very specific, realistic goals. You know what fitness factors you need to address. You know how to measure them. You're almost there. All that's left is to determine sensible

If you're not sure where you're going, you'll probably end up nowhere.

goals and how to trick yourself into sticking with them this time. Here's how.

Determine a starting point and an ending point. You've already done most of the work if you've gone through the evaluation process. Let's say you check in at 30 percent body fat. That's your starting point. You also know your ending point. If you're a woman, to stay in what experts consider the "healthy" range means having no more than 26 percent body fat. This is much more precise than picking an arbitrary number of pounds to lose, since you don't know how much of those pounds will be fat or lean body tissue. Record the starting point and ending point with each of the five fitness factors. If your goals are more athletic, you'll need to modify the procedure a bit. If you wish to complete a 5-mile race in 40 minutes, find out how fast you can run that distance now. Just make sure your goals are within the realm of possibility. No one has ever run 5 miles in less than 20 minutes.

Set both short-term and long-term goals. It's good to have a large, ultimate goal but you may get discouraged if it takes months to reach it. Smaller, stepping-stone goals help keep you interested and serve as checkpoints along the way, letting you know you're headed in the right direction. To go from 30 to 20 per-

cent body fat, you might break it up into five 2 percent mini-goals.

Map out your routine. You have your goals. Now put them into action. Take a few minutes to design an eating and exercise routine. You should know how many days a week you plan to do aerobic exercises, lift weights, or skip dessert. Have a general idea of how much time you intend to spend exercising and the type and intensity of each workout. You can always set aside some time for spontaneity as long as the major details are there. Write it all down. Your goals, your plan, everything. Then keep a workout diary. If you succeed and achieve your goals, you'll have a written record of exactly what works for you. If you don't hit your mark, review what you've been doing and make changes.

Have a backup plan. Sometimes you get sidetracked and lose sight of your goals. So it's always good to have a plan B. If you get injured and can't run, you could continue working toward a better flexibility score while you heal. If you get injured and can't masturbate, then you've got problems. In any case, try to avoid the "all or nothing" mentality. It steers most people straight into nothing. Anything is better than nothing.

Personalize it. Bottom line: you won't get very far if you don't like what you're

none of yer beeswax

Psychological studies show that the most embarrassing question to ask a person isn't about sex. It's "What do you weigh?"

It's possible that you'll trim 5 pounds a year or prevent a 5-pound gain by burning just 50 extra calories a day. By doing at least one of these activities daily, you'll use up extra calories without even trying. This is based on a 135-pound person, by the way.

Light housework, like dusting, ironing, or scooping up kitty dung	20 minutes
Golf in a foursome (wearing clothes)	14 minutes
Mowing the lawn with a hand-pushed power mower	13 minutes
Brisk walk to the store, massage parlor, or away from crime scene	12 minutes
Romantic slow dance or slow, pulsating, throbbing sex	11 minutes
Vacuuming, scrubbing floors, or bonding with your erotic partner	10 minutes
Gardening, clipping bushes, or burying evidence	9 minutes
Climbing stairs or climbing the walls	7.5 minutes
Shoveling snow, hay, or horse manure	5.5 minutes

doing or it doesn't fit into your schedule. Choose activities you enjoy. Eat healthy foods you like. Figure out how much time you can spare for your workouts. You can always split it up if you don't have one big block of time. If you don't get it right on your first go-round, try again. There's something for everyone.

Results May Vary

Models, ironically, are not good role models. Most women can't achieve a 36-inch bust and 18-inch waist without massive surgical retooling. Yet it's the genetic freaks that end up on magazine covers and runways, somehow making the rest of us feel like genetic freaks. Men's expectations aren't usually any more realistic, though they don't seem to stress out about it as much as women do. Still, most of them don't have a genetic chance in hell of ending up on the side of a bus in their underwear. Trying to achieve a look that doesn't mesh with your body type is counterproductive. Playing up your natural assets is much more empowering.

It takes all morphs. So now that you've figured out how in or out of shape you are, what kind of eater you are, how much fat you have, how muscular you are, and exactly which kind of morph you are, you can use the following chapters to

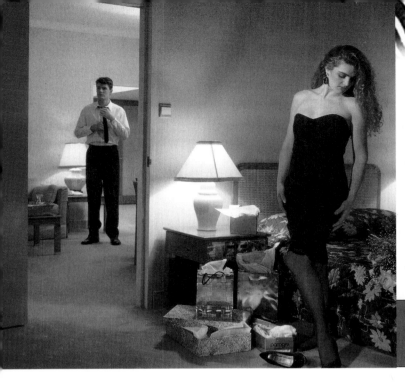

take measures to sculpt it, enhance it, change it, or ignore it altogether and just get healthy. And don't get too obsessed about this morph thing. It's just to help you learn about your body so that you can work out smarter and get better results without wasting a lot of time. Maybe we all wish we could be mesomorphs, but if we were, life wouldn't be nearly as interesting and suddenly all of us seemingly perfect mesomorphs would want to be endomorphs. You have learned your fitness test results and your true body type and you know what to do with it. So pack your morph into some workout gear and let's learn the strength-training exercises that can help you sculpt that genetically inherited frame of yours.

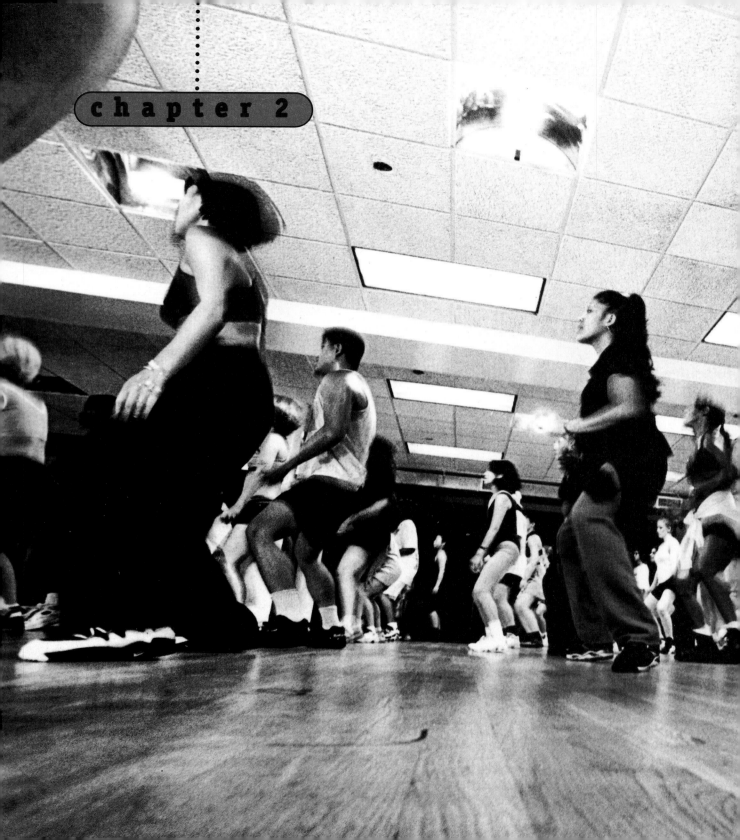

move!

Heart and Soul, Frying Calories, and the Joy of Aerobics

Jane Fonda Didn't Invent Aerobics

Aerobics weren't invented by Jane Fonda, although the term "aerobic" was first used in the late sixties—about the same time the Queen of Lean was practicing "nude aerobics" in the screen marvel *Barbarella.* About the same time the Beatles were practicing "popularity aerobics" running from screaming, obsessed horny teen girls. And about the same time Mr. Nixon was doing "peace-sign waving" aerobics running for President. While the term wasn't officially coined until 1968 by a physician named Dr. Kenneth Cooper, aerobics have been in full swing since Fred and Barney were chasing after brontosaurus burgers.

Aerobic means, literally, "with air." When you move your larger muscle groups, like your arms and legs, in a steady and rhythmic fashion over an extended period of time, your working muscles require more oxygen, contained in the air you breathe, to continue functioning. The harder your body works, the harder your cardiovascular system works ("cardio" means heart and blood vessels) and the harder your lungs work to keep up with your body's oxygen demands.

HOW DO WE TALK OURSELVES OUT OF EXERCISING?

It's not your brain—it's smart enough to know why you should get moving. It's not your heart—which desperately needs you to exercise. It's not your stomach . . . it just comes along for the ride. Guess who wants you to stay seated? Guess who's most comfortable not moving? Guess who doesn't worry about getting in shape thanks to muumuus, X-large jeans, long blazers, tunics, and skirts? Guess who never gets truly unhealthy (just flabby), like the heart, when you don't exercise? That's right pal. It's your ass . . .

As a lazy ass, I hate exercise books. They should write a book like *Techniques for Sitting on Your Ass for Hours.*

That's why your heart rate (number of times your heart beats per minute) increases and you take faster, deeper breaths when you exercise.

If you put your body through its aerobic paces often enough, some lasting physical changes occur. While you're at rest, your heart beats slower and pumps out more blood per stroke because it's stronger and more efficient. Your lungs, now able to suck in more air, become more proficient at extracting oxygen from the air you take in. Things you used to find difficult, like climbing stairs, hitting golf balls in your yard at 11 P.M., or a ménage à trois with the Cirque de Soleil, suddenly seem easier.

Burning Calories and Fat

Now, this life-sustaining, disease-preventing stuff is all well and good, but enough about why the hypocrites work out. For most of us vanity is more often the driving factor for why we do what we do. We want to be thinner, more attractive. We want to look good in clothes and at least passable in a bathing suit. Luckily aerobic exercise can help with that too. We've already mentioned that aerobic exercise burns fat and calories. There's also an indication that it revs up your metabolism even when you're not exercising,

causing a slight calorie afterburn for hours after a workout. Yet aerobic exercise is most effective when combined with strength training. So, while aerobic exercise diminishes slow-metabolizing body fat, strength training increases fast-metabolizing lean body tissue. Add a low-fat eating plan and you have an unbeatable weight control combination.

You may have also heard that the best way to lose weight is to aerobicize at a very slow steady pace for a long duration, which puts you into what has been dubbed the fat-burning zone. During long, slow aerobic workouts, the theory goes, your body gets its fuel in the form of fat, derived from a substance in your bloodstream scientists call free fatty acids. When you push yourself to work at a faster pace, your body relies on a greater percentage of glycogen—your body's largest carbohydrate reserve—for energy.

> Medical studies show that only aerobic and resistance exercise burns fat and that fat-burning pills only burn cash.

Conclusion? Since lower-intensity exercise uses more fat, it's the most effective way to burn off body fat.

While it's true you rely on a greater percentage of fat during lower-intensity exercise, you burn a certain percentage of all fuels at all intensities. The proportion of calories you burn from fat is fairly small when you're working harder, but the total number you burn from fat is higher.

Let's say you walk 30 minutes at a speed that isn't very taxing and cover 1.5 miles. If you're 135 pounds, you'll burn 106 calories, about 80 percent or 84 calories from fat. Let's say you run 30 minutes and double the distance. You'll burn around 330 calories, and even if only 50 percent are derived from fat, you'll burn a total number of 170 fat calories. The workout that uses the most calories contributes the most to weight loss. A calorie burned is a calorie burned, no matter how you fry the little suckers. That means you can go for broke and push yourself to the limit or, if you're not in the mood or not ready for a high-octane workout, you can stroll along and enjoy the scenery. Or you may want to mix it up and do what we call "wave training," in which you fluctuate between varying intensities during a workout.

Julie says . . .

ALWAYS WARM UP BEFORE EXERCISING . . .

A good warm-up is any activity that wakes your body up, and warms up your muscles and mind for more strenuous activity. It can prevent injuries and stress to your heart. You also feel better during your workout when you get into it slowly.

In case you didn't know, a warm-up means movement, not stretching. Marching in place, walking briskly, pedaling on a stationary bicycle for 5 minutes are all you really need to warm up muscles and get the blood going. It's always a good idea to do at least a little of this before you stretch; stretching a "cold" muscle can lead to muscle pulls and really isn't as effective as stretching a muscle that has a little warmth and blood flow.

Most experts will tell you to save your stretching for the end of your workout to help you cool down (see the chapter "Stretch!" beginning on page 143).

Talk the Talk as You Walk

So how do you know if you're working hard enough to consider what you're doing aerobic? There are lots of ways to tell, starting with the "huff and puff" factor. If you're breathless and can't carry on even snatches of a conversation, you're overdoing it and need to slow down until you can speak in breathy, but complete sentences. If you're slogging along belting out the words to "Tonight's the Night" with Rod Stewart, you need to pick up the pace. Obviously this "talk test," though useful, isn't a very exact science. A much more

comfortable?

For every home gym, there are 15,423 La-Z-Boys.

precise method of measuring exercise intensity involves tracking your heart rate.

Your Target Training Zone
Easier to find than the G-spot (but not as much fun).

As we've already told you, when you exercise, your heart has to pump harder and faster in order to keep pace with your body's greater demand for blood and oxygen. That's why tracking your heart rate is such a good indicator of exercise intensity.

For you browser-type readers, see the box on page 28 for a quick rundown on how fast your heart should beat—based on your age, conditioning, and goals—during a typical workout. But for those able to resist immediate gratification, first let's talk about your maximum heart rate and how to determine your proper "target training zone."

To get an estimate of your "age-predicted" maximum heart rate, subtract your age from 220 if you're a man and from 226 if you're a woman. Theoretically, this number is the fastest your heart is capable of beating no matter what, even if you were to spend several hours trying to drag all six friends out of that coffee bar; through research, experts have discovered that the average person's maximum declines about one beat each year. This age-predicted maximum heart rate formula requires nothing more than your true age and a grasp of simple arithmetic, but there are other, more accurate ways to get a portrait of what your cardiovascular system is capable of; a doctor or physiologist can perform tests to determine a precise, personalized maximum based on your fitness level rather than your age. It's not absolutely necessary, but if you're curious, or if you've had health problems, you might want to consider a visit to a professional. And, of course, if you're training for a hard-core athletic event, it's a good idea to see a physiologist or doctor anyway. Just know that if you figure your age-predicted max, it can be off by as much as 15 beats.

During exercise, you want your heart rate to be higher than it is at rest and below your maximum. We call this your target training zone, also known as your target heart rate, your target heart zone, or your THZ. Your target training zone falls anywhere between 50 and 90 percent of your maximum heart rate. To figure it out, simply multiply your maximum heart rate by 0.5 and 0.9. Write those two numbers down, and the next time you exercise, take your pulse and see if your heartbeat falls somewhere in between. Staying within your target training zone prevents you from either going overboard or dogging it.

How to Take Your Heart Rate

Place two fingers on your wrist directly below the base of your thumb, feel for the thumping of your pulse, and count how many times your heart beats in 15 seconds. Multiply this number by 4 and you get how many times your heart beats per minute. You should take your heart rate every 20 minutes or so, more often if you're new to aerobic exercise. Never use your thumb to take your pulse since your thumb has a pulse of its own. If you have trouble finding the pulse at your wrist try sliding your fingers into the groove on either side of your Adam's apple instead. Just don't press too hard because this may artificially slow your heart rate and give you the impression you're not working as hard as you really are; it can also make you feel faint. You may also want to use a heart rate monitor that straps around your chest and sends your heart rate readings to a special wristwatch; this is the easiest and most accurate method of tracking your heart rate short of hard-wiring yourself into a physician's medical ECG unit.

Now that you're skilled at touching yourself in special places, you'll be able to control your heart rate with reasonable precision. You'll know exactly how hard you need to work to stay within your zone. At that point, you can begin refining your larger, overall zone into a series of mini-zones. Rather than looking to work within that broad, 50–90 percent range, you might want to exercise within the 80–90 percent range to get a harder workout or stay closer to the 50 percent if you want an easier one. Depending on your current condition and what you're trying to accomplish, you'll spend more time in some mini-zones than in others. Once you learn how various exercise routines affect your heart rate, you'll be able to fluctuate between mini-zones at will, similar to the ability to pee loudly to impress or softly to be discreet. We call this multiple training zone approach "wave training." It's featured in detail on the following pages; take a look to determine which zone or zones you should be spending your time in.

THE SIX BRAINLESS STEPS TO FIGURING OUT YOUR HEART RATE AND TARGET TRAINING ZONE

1. While moving, place two fingers on wrist pulse point.
2. Count how many thumps you feel in 15 seconds.
3. This number times 4 = heartbeats per minute.
4. Rate should increase until it reaches target training zone or 50–90 percent of your maximum heart rate.
5. Maximum heart rate = 220 minus your age for men, 226 minus your age for women.
6. Multiply your maximum heart rate times 0.5 and 0.9 to see if you fall within your target training zone.

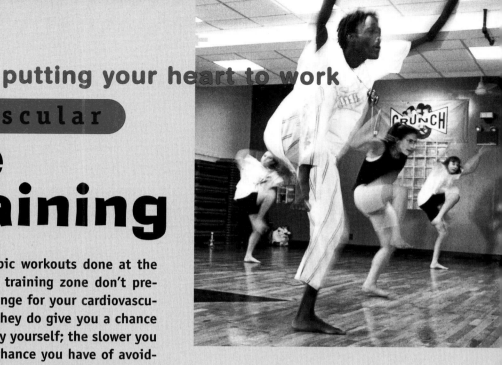

cardiovascular
wave training

Long, slow aerobic workouts done at the low end of your training zone don't present a big challenge for your cardiovascular system, but they do give you a chance to relax and enjoy yourself; the slower you go, the greater chance you have of avoiding injury too. Moderately hard workouts increase your odds of injury and overtraining yet offer greater aerobic benefits. Shorter, higher-intensity training sessions develop your anaerobic energy systems, which rely on chemicals stored in your muscles, rather than just oxygen, for energy. Your anaerobic system is responsible for short, powerful bursts of movement like dashing across the tennis court and chasing the jerk who goosed your girlfriend. Anaerobic levels can only be sustained briefly and may be too extreme for less experienced exercisers.

Wave training uses five training zones rather than one. This helps you take advantage of changes in intensity while minimizing the disadvantages of staying at one end of a wide-ranging zone all the time. Each training zone is based on a narrow range of heart rates, your goals, and, of course, your fitness level:

Zone One
(50–60 percent of maximum heart rate)

You're relaxed, trotting along. Your breathing is regular, steady, and a bit deeper than it is at rest. To help prevent injuries and soreness, beginners should do the bulk of their workouts in the moderate zone for at least a month or until they feel ready for more intense workouts. This zone is suited for slow workouts lasting 60 minutes or more—like walking on a flat surface or a very slow jog.

Zone Two
(60–70 percent of maximum heart rate)

Though still comfortable, your breathing is deeper. You're moving at a good, but not killer, clip. This zone is ideal for 30–60-minute workouts: jogging, skating, or swimming. It's good for beginners ready to push harder—you can crisscross intervals using this and the moderate zone.

Zone Three
(70–80 percent of maximum heart rate)

Your breathing is stronger and heavier, as your lungs have really kicked into gear. Your pace is very challenging but still doable. This may be too strenuous for beginning exercisers to do for more than brief intervals, but ideal for advanced exercisers doing up to 30 minutes of cardiovascular training. Examples: intense aerobic dance, jogging or cycling on hills. To increase your stamina and strength, do at least two full workouts a week that take you into this zone for at least ten minutes.

Zone Four
(80–90 percent of maximum heart rate)

Your breathing is quick and sharp, your heart is pounding, and your muscles fatigue quickly when you train at this level. You'll need to stop completely or move very slowly between anaerobic threshold intervals. Several 2–10-minute intervals at this level once or twice a week helps advanced exercisers develop speed and power. You can run or cycle up a steep hill.

Zone Five
(90–100 percent of maximum heart rate —yikes)

This is your all-out, Go Speed Racer pace. Breathing is choppy. Your heart feels like it's going to jump out of your chest. For brief intervals lasting no more than 60 seconds, and only if you're extremely fit and peaking for competition. Examples: sprinting or cycling up very steep hills.

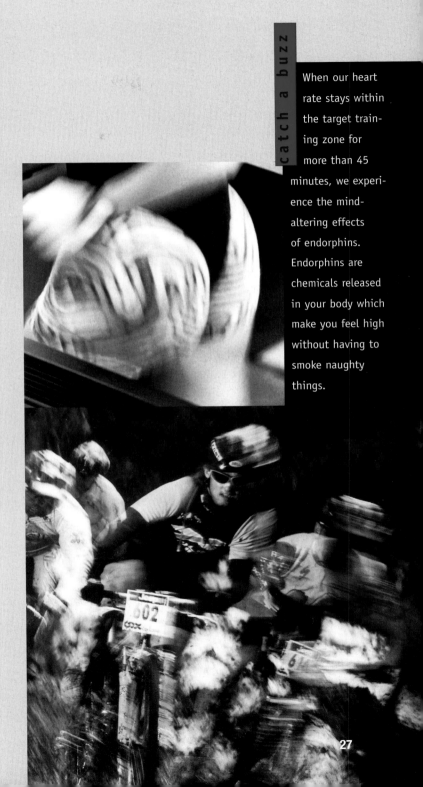

catch a buzz

When our heart rate stays within the target training zone for more than 45 minutes, we experience the mind-altering effects of endorphins. Endorphins are chemicals released in your body which make you feel high without having to smoke naughty things.

age	heart rate zone one	heart rate zone two	heart rate zone three	heart rate zone four	heart rate zone five
	50%–60%	60%–70%	70%–80%	80%–90% threshold	90%–100%
20	100–120	120–140	140–160	160–180	180–200
25	98–117	117–137	137–156	156–175	175–195
30	95–114	114–133	133–152	152–171	171–190
35	93–111	111–130	130–148	148–166	166–185
40	90–108	108–126	126–144	144–162	162–180
45	88–105	105–123	123–140	140–158	158–175
50	85–102	102–119	119–136	136–153	153–170
55	83–99	99–116	116–132	132–149	149–165
60	80–96	96–112	112–128	128–144	144–160
65	78–93	93–109	109–124	124–140	140–155

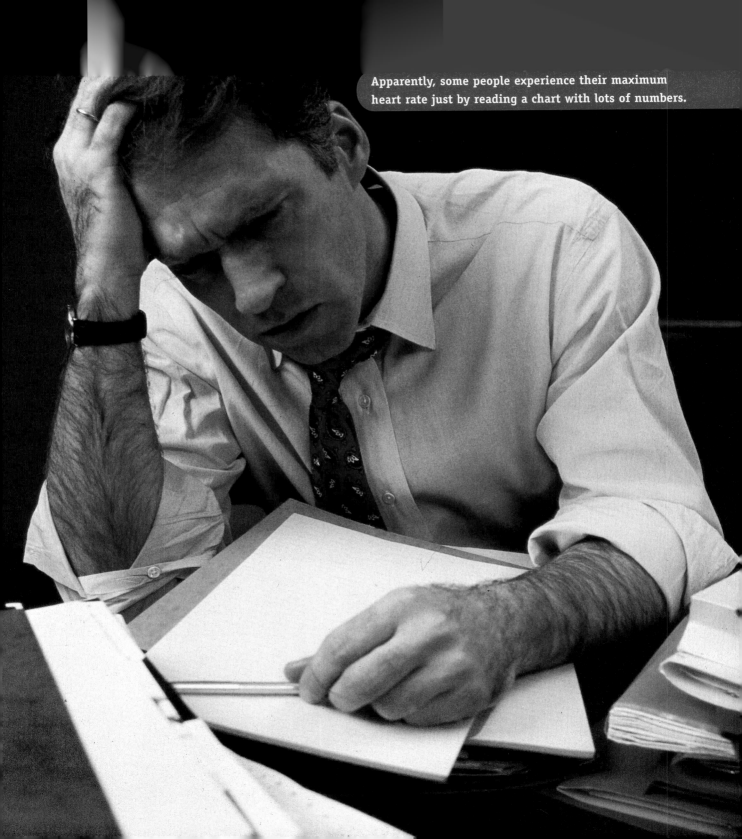

Apparently, some people experience their maximum heart rate just by reading a chart with lots of numbers.

Math homework's done and you have your handy heart rate chart. Now what? First, you need to decide why you should even do anything when you're perfectly comfortable on the couch. That question alone may be enough to send your heart into its target training zone. . . . Luckily there are loopholes in the logic of lazy. It's easy. You just have to choose which program fits your lifestyle, personality, preferences, and any weird pet peeves or phobias you might have. If treadmills, for instance, remind you of the pointlessness and futility of life, avoid them. You need to choose a program you'll enjoy and stick with. Here's a rundown on some of the most tried-and-true aerobic alternatives.

Top Aerobic Exercises

Walking

The Scoop

It's the most natural activity you can call exercise. Though walkers burn a lot fewer calories per minute than, say, joggers and in-line skaters, most people last longer on a walk than a run, so it evens out. Walking doesn't involve a lot of pounding but it

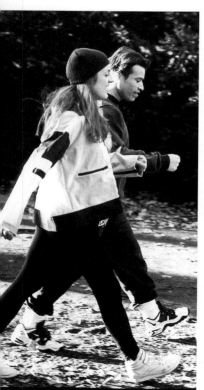

does involve a lot of muscles, so it's a good way to tone up without a high incidence of injury.

The trouble is, many people find walking to be a lot like, well . . . walking, which is boring. You think, "How can something people can do in their sleep make me someone more people will want to sleep with?" Excellent question. Well, there are lots of ways to pump up your walking program. Read on and we'll tell you all about 'em.

Just When You Thought You Knew How to Walk

The biggest mistake walkers make is not standing up straight. The universe's punishment for slouchers can be problems in your lower back, neck, and hips: your posture should be naturally tall. Relax your shoulders, widen your chest, and pull your abdominals gently inward. Keep your head and chin up, and focus straight ahead. Keep your hands relaxed and cupped gently, and swing your arms so they brush past your body. On the upswing, your hand should be level with your breast bone; on the downswing, your hand should brush against your hip. Keep your hips loose and relaxed. Your feet should land firmly, heel first. Roll through your heel to your arch, then to the ball of your foot, then to your toes. Push off from your toes and ball of your foot.

Now drop and give me fifty, you pathetic little . . . Sorry, anyway, most people walk with basically good form right from the start; they just need a few reminders. It's a good idea to run through a mental head-to-toe checklist every so often to see how you're doing.

Essential Gear

You can walk in your business suit or in your birthday suit, it really doesn't matter. As long as your feet are well shod you should be able to avoid knee, hip, and lower-back problems. A good pair of walking shoes will run you at least $40; look for shoes that are flexible, because your feet bend when you walk. They should have lots of cushioning too—especially around the ball of the foot—because you push off your toes with quite a bit of oomph. Also, since your heels bear most of your weight when you walk, you need a firm, stable heel counter. That's the part of the shoe that wraps around your heel to keep your foot anchored in place. Walking shoes should hold up for 1,000 to 1,500 miles; replace them when the tread begins to wear thin or when the sides start to cave inward or outward.

Tips for Rookies

If you don't have time for a formalized workout, sneak in a walk whenever you can. Take a 15-minute walk during your lunch break. Walk to the store every time you're out of milk instead of driving the six blocks. Park at the far corner of the parking lot (as long as it's safe). Just make sure you go fast enough to stay in your target training zone heart rate to get the full cardiovascular effect.

Besides, the faster you walk, the more calories you burn. If you walk very fast—at a 12-minute-mile to 15-minute-mile pace—you burn twice as many calories as when you walk at a typical, strolling 20-minute-mile pace. If you move very, very fast—so fast you have to hold yourself back from breaking into a run—walking burns more calories than running. You might want to leave that kind of walking to the professionals until you're a little more comfortable with this one-foot-in-front-of-the-other thing, but as you get in shape, you can mix in some fast-paced intervals.

Another way to spice up your walking program—get off the beaten track. Take a hike. Hit the trails. Walk over hilly, rugged terrain. It'll shape your buttocks and thighs even more and help burn extra calories. A 135-pound person walking a mile over flat terrain will burn about a 100 calories, but if she walks the same distance over a modestly hilly course, she'll double the calorie burn.

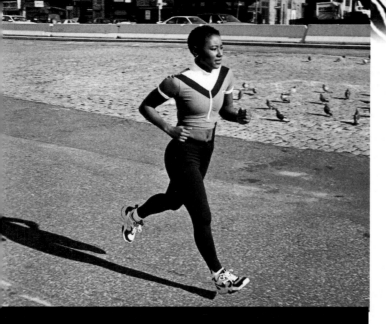

Running

The Scoop

Like walking, running is a portable workout which requires the minimum of equipment. It burns lots of calories and leaves your muscles feeling pleasantly worked. Running and jogging don't require much concentration and may help you slip into a calmer mental state similar to dreaming and meditation—a state of mind which many experts feel is ideal for creative thinking, problem solving, and easing stress. Runners reverently refer to this as a "runner's high."

On the downside, runners tend to have frequent, chronic injuries. Many people have joints that simply will not tolerate all that pounding—up to two times your body weight per stride. If you're not built to run, don't fight it. There are unlimited ways to get in great condition. If you're one of

Beginning Runners Chart

Running for 30 consecutive minutes can be a bit much when you're first starting out. Try this three-times-a-week routine for the first four weeks of training, then gradually reduce your walking intervals as you lengthen your running intervals. Eventually, you'll be able to run the entire 30 minutes.

walk/run workout 1	walk/run workout 2	walk/run workout 3
walk 5 minutes easy	walk 5 minutes easy	walk 1 minute easy
walk 3 minutes moderate-fast	walk 2 minutes moderate-fast	walk 2 minutes moderate-fast
run 3 minutes easy	run 5 minutes easy	run 4 minutes easy
walk 3 minutes moderate-fast	walk 2 minutes moderate-fast	walk 4 minutes moderate-fast
run 3 minutes easy	run 5 minutes easy	run 4 minutes easy
walk 5 minutes moderate-easy	walk 5 minutes easy-moderate	walk 4 minutes easy-moderate
run 2 minutes easy	run 2 minutes easy	run 6 minutes easy
walk 3 minutes fast	walk 2 minutes fast	walk 3 minutes fast
walk 3 minutes easy	walk 2 minutes easy	walk 2 minutes easy
TOTAL WALK: 22 MINUTES	**TOTAL WALK: 18 MINUTES**	**TOTAL WALK: 16 MINUTES**
TOTAL RUN: 8 MINUTES	**TOTAL RUN: 12 MINUTES**	**TOTAL RUN: 14 MINUTES**
TOTAL TIME: 30 MINUTES	**TOTAL TIME: 30 MINUTES**	**TOTAL TIME: 30 MINUTES**

those pathological runners (what are you running from?), try mixing it in with a bunch of other cross-training activities. Resistance training to strengthen knees and ankles is another way to help prevent injuries.

Good Stuff to Know

Runners have this habit of looking directly at the ground, maybe looking for dropped money to help them buy more running stuff. This throws your upper-body posture off kilter and can lead to upper-back and neck pain. Make sure you keep your head lifted and your eyes focused straight ahead. Keep your shoulders relaxed, your chest open, and your abdominal muscles pulled in tightly. Don't arch your back excessively; that's one of the main reasons runners get back and hip pain. Keep your arms bent at a 90-degree angle and hold them close to your body. Swing them forward and back rather than across your body, and don't clench your fists. Don't shuffle along like you're wearing boots. Lift your front knee and extend your back leg. Let your feet do the work, not your shoes. Land heel first and roll through the entire length of your foot. Push off from the balls of your feet, instead of running flat-footed and pounding off your heels.

Essential Gear

Running clothes aren't just for runners anymore. If looking like a runner and feeling like a runner makes you feel like running, then you're really motivated by your wardrobe, and that's okay. However, the only equipment that's truly essential for running is a good pair of shoes. (Though larger-breasted women may want to wear a good sports bra to prevent bouncing.)

The shoe that's best for you depends on your weight, the shape of your foot, your running style, and any joint problems you may have, such as weak ankles or bad knees. Try to buy your running shoes at a shop that specializes in running gear and get the help of an experienced salesperson. Once you find out what works for you, you may be able to get them cheaper through catalogs or generalized sporting-goods stores.

Expect to fork over between $60 and $100 for a decent pair of running shoes. Your running shoes should be fairly flexible, especially across the ball of the foot. When you go into a store, hold the shoe on both ends and bend it; it should break right at the ball of the foot. You want cushioning, but not so much that you can't feel your foot hitting the ground. Look for stable heel counters. If your foot slides around a lot, that can quite literally mean trouble down the road somewhere.

An unfortunate fact about running shoes is that the manufacturers feel the need to change their design frequently, probably to justify the existence of their marketing department. You'll probably find a brand and a model that you like a lot, only to have it phased out for something touted as "new and better" which totally doesn't work for you. Once you find a shoe you like, stockpile a couple of pairs or be prepared to renew your search for a decent running shoe every year or so.

Tips for Rookies

Start by alternating periods of walking with periods of running. Two minutes walking, one minute running is a good place to start. Gradually decrease your walking intervals until you can run continuously for 20 minutes and build from there. To avoid injuries, don't increase your mileage by more than 10 percent a week. Also, take at least one day off from running each week.

Even after you phase out walking, vary your pace. Don't always drag along barely lifting your feet but don't try to sprint all out every time out either. Different paces work your heart, lungs, and legs in different ways. Plus, the variety makes running more fun. Races can satisfy the competitive urge. We're not just talking major marathons here. Most people find training for a local 10K or informal "fun run" enough to keep them focused and challenged.

Swimming

The Scoop

More than 13 percent of the population swims every day. Perhaps that's because water's cushioning effects make swimming an ideal "body-friendly" aerobic choice, great for people with joint problems and people trying to avoid joint problems. Because water resists your action in any direction you move, it offers a "3-D" strengthening effect. So, say you do a bench press type of movement like the one on page 70. If you do this exercise in the gym or at home, you strengthen your chest muscles as you straighten your arms but you pretty much get a free ride as you bend your arms back to the start. When you do the same movement in water, you feel resistance, in the form of water pressure, on the upward movement *and* the downward movement, so both your chest and back muscles get a workout. That's why swimming builds muscle strength and tone so evenly.

Another big advantage to swimming—or any activity you do in the water—is that a little extra body fat works in your favor. It helps you glide along near the surface of the water, so you don't expend a lot of frustrated energy trying to keep yourself from sinking like a stone. In other words, your seat may be used as a flotation device.

Yup, swimming gets high ratings in just about every way you can think of. Except where weight loss is concerned. Unfortunately, research seems to indicate that it isn't the best way to drop body fat, possibly because your heart can't pump as fast as it does during land-based activities and possibly because cool water temperatures may put the brakes on fat loss. However, some new studies suggest that one of the reasons swimming isn't very helpful in the weight loss department is that most people don't work at it very hard. If you push yourself a little, you'll increase both calorie and fat burn. Keep at it for a while and good technique and strong upper-body muscles will help you swim farther, faster.

Good Stuff to Know

As we told you, it's harder to get your heart rate up when you swim. You should still strive to get in your target heart zone, but in the water this zone will be 10 to 12 beats lower than usual. You'll also need to rethink your whole concept of distance. A mile of swimming can take an inexperienced swimmer over an hour to complete.

Essential Gear

It depends on where you swim, but in most places swimsuits are not optional. By the way, we said swimsuit, not bathing suit. You don't want something that looks pretty when you're on display at the beach but keeps creeping up your butt or slipping off your shoulders.

If you swim in a chlorinated pool, goggles are a must to prevent eye irritation. Cheap goggles—$5 to $10—tend to be just as good as the $40 kind. Buy them at a swim store that allows you to try them on. You should feel some suction around your eyes, but not so much that you feel like your eyeballs are being sucked out. You also need a cap. Sure, you may feel like you're wearing a condom on your head. You are. It *prevents* your hair from getting in your face when you swim and *protects* your hair from harsh chemicals. Most pools require them for anyone with longer than ear-length hair anyway.

As for all those fun swimming gadgets you see lined up on the edge of pools: Most pools let you borrow the equipment, but you can buy a whole set, including rubber swimming fins, a pull buoy, and a kickboard, for less than $100. All of these help you concentrate on different aspects of your form. Swimming with a pull buoy between your legs, for instance, allows you to isolate your upper body; holding on to a kickboard allows you to perfect your kick. You might also want to invest in a pair of plastic hand paddles, which are slightly larger than your hand.

When wearing paddles, it takes more strength to complete each stroke, so your upper body gets an extra challenge.

Tips for Rookies

Even if you're in good aerobic shape from doing other things, you'll probably feel out of breath the first few times you swim. Be patient. You're body will acclimate soon enough to the specific demands swimming places on it. Start out with a total of 15–20 minutes accumulated swim time and give yourself the okay to take frequent rest breaks. Concentrate on your technique and form; most people need a lesson or two to help them master the basic strokes (the crawl, backstroke, butterfly, and breaststroke). The better your technique, the easier time you'll have propelling yourself through water so you'll reap the full cardio and muscle effects.

Swimming isn't the only way to get wet during a workout by the way. Check out an aqua running or water aerobics class at your local pool. Wild and wacky offerings like aqua yoga and underwater stepping may also appeal to you.

Cycling

The Scoop

Many ex-runners turn to cycling when their joints can't take being beaten to a pulp any longer but exercising in water holds no at- traction; other types of people gravitate toward cycling too. It's not hard to learn, provides a decent aerobic workout, tones your legs and butt muscles, and promotes coordination and balance. Cycling is also a good way to see the sights, because you can cover a lot of ground quickly—you can go two or three times the distance on a bike than you can on foot.

Cycling does have its negatives, however. For one thing, you need a truckload of equipment. (We'll fill you in on that shortly.) For another, your chances of taking a header are pretty good. Car accidents resulting in head injuries are the number one injury to cyclists; about half a million cyclists visit the emergency room each year.

Good Stuff to Know

Always wear a helmet when you cycle in case you fall. Ride with traffic rather than against it, avoiding heavily traveled highways when you can. Follow the rules of the road. This means stopping at *all* stop signs and using those hand turn signals you learned in driver's ed. Never assume the driver sees you, even if he appears to be staring you down. Carry a tool kit and learn how to fix a flat tire, so you don't end up giving your bike a lift home.

Knee pain is the next most common injury after being tossed into traffic; it's of-

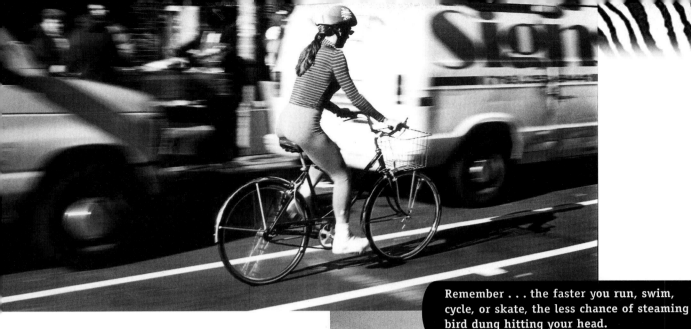

ten the result of an incorrect seat setting. Correct seating means that in the fully extended position your knee should be slightly bent but not completely locked. Back pain, another common cyclist complaint, may be the result of staying in a hunched-over position for too long; if you feel pain coming on, get off and take a break. A regular strengthening and stretching program will help you sidestep these types of injuries.

Essential Gear

If you haven't shopped for a bike since the ninth grade, prepare yourself for sticker shock. Even a basic 10-speed (which is now 14–16 speeds, by the way) is going to set you back at least a couple of hundred dollars; many are priced closer to the $1,000 range. You don't need to go top-of-the-line but if you're serious about get-

ting into cycling, you don't want to go el cheapo either.

Most people nowadays, about 80 percent, opt for a mountain bike, a bike category that didn't even exist ten years ago. Built for abuse, they're the pit bull of the biking world, with wide, fat tires and upright handlebars. They're more comfortable and more versatile—you can ride on dirt trails, through puddles, and over potholes in the pavement. But they're also clunky and slow. If you plan to cover long distances quickly and stay on the road, you're better off with a multigeared road bike with skinny tires and curved handlebars, similar to the one you rode as a kid. A third option is a hybrid, which is basically a heavy road bike with upright handlebars and a cushy saddle. Hybrids are good for tooling around town, but they're annoyingly slow for long-distance road riding and very limiting on mountain trails.

Besides the actual bike itself, a bike helmet is absolutely essential gear; light but sturdy ones are made especially for biking. Cycling gloves, sunglasses, and a water bottle are also standard must-have items; special clothing like shorts with a padded behind and a shirt with a large pouch sewn into the back for storing a snack or an extra T-shirt are also things that make for a comfortable ride. By the time you're done looking like a cyclist, don't be surprised if your Visa bill is looking like a mountain.

Tips for Rookies

Although cycling doesn't impact your joints like other sports, it still can be hard on your body. You'll still feel achy and sore, especially your legs and butt muscles. You can minimize some of the soreness by starting out slowly (as with any exercise activity) and pedaling at the proper cadence. Cadence refers to the number of revolutions per minute that you pedal. Inexperienced cyclists tend to pedal in a tighter gear than they can handle, which forces them into a slow cadence; their legs tire prematurely and they cheat themselves out of a good workout. Try to train at a cadence of 90 to 100 r.p.m., which means pedaling quickly with fairly light tension (most bikes have a speedometer which indicates both miles per hour and r.p.m.s).

When you do go off-road, start on wide dirt roads rather than narrow "single track" trails that require technical skill. (And don't think that because there are no cars, you're immune from injury.) Mountain biking is great for building leg strength, but if you spend all your time negotiating obstacles and carrying your bike over ditches and streams, you won't get an aerobic workout. Try to spend at least 60 percent of your time on the road or perhaps on a stationary bike doing some steady, uninterrupted cardiovascular training.

Skating
The Scoop

Here's another thing that's evolved into something more than it was when you were a pimple-faced teen. The skates you used to rent at the roller rink, the kind with a pair of wheels at the toe and a pair of wheels at the heel, have been superseded by skates on which the wheels are positioned in a straight line down the center of the boot. When this "in-line" skate was introduced in 1980 by Rollerblade, Inc., it caused a skate revolution. Now more than 15 million Americans own in-line skates.

Skating is fun because it isn't as straight-ahead as running, walking, and cycling. You can curve, turn, glide, sprint, and spin. It's definitely aerobic too, burning almost as many calories as jogging. Stopping, turning, and skating backward all enhance balance, agility, and coordination. It's also one of the few aerobic activities that strengthen and tone the hard-to-reach inner and outer thigh muscles. Go skating often enough and don't be surprised when you end up with skater's butt, skater's legs, skater's abs, and skater's upper body. (All good things.)

Good Stuff to Know

Safety is a big issue with skating: one in 150 skaters takes a trip to the emergency room each year. Even though it's considered a low-impact workout (meaning it doesn't place much stress on the joints), when you fall, believe us—you'll impact. Skaters often put out their hands to break a fall, which can result in wrist fractures. Abrasions, head injuries, twisted ankles, and banged-up knees are other common skating injuries, all a result of falling. A lesson or two is definitely a good idea, because the pavement will cushion your fall the same way a bus, a tree, or a statue of a soldier holding a bayonet does. Most skate shops have pros available for group or private lessons.

Essential Gear

You'll find that in-line skates have more advantages over conventional roller skates than just wheel

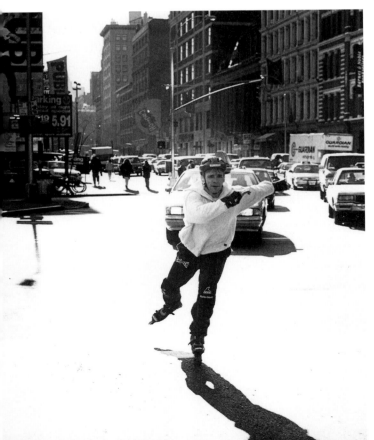

use your head

More than 30,000 in-line skaters visit emergency rooms each year. 31.7 percent wear no protective gear at all. Only 2 percent wear helmets.

placement. The wheels are faster, smoother, and more durable. And the boots are made of lightweight nylon rather than thick leather, so they breathe more easily and conform to your feet much better. You'll spend between $100 and $400 for good in-lines.

Try on several pairs at the store, and wear each for *at least* 10 minutes, until your feet start to get hot. Tilt your feet to the inside and the outside, putting plenty of pressure on your foot to make sure nothing hurts. Otherwise, you're asking for blisters. The boots should feel snug in the toe and heel. If your heel is loose, you won't have enough control when you skate.

A helmet is as essential for skating as it is for biking. A cycling helmet will suffice, but they do make special in-line helmets with more protection at the rear of the head. Also crucial: wrist guards, knee guards, elbow guards (about $20 each or $30 to $50 for a pack that contains all three). A good way to stay intact is to buy safety gear *before* you buy skates so you won't be tempted to take them for an unprotected test drive.

Tips for Rookies

Experienced skaters make it look easy, but gliding along with effortless grace takes practice. Beginners should work on stopping techniques first; then turning, cornering, downhill skating, and staying upright. Learn to balance by walking on the skates on your living-room carpet or your lawn. Then head to a parking lot to practice skating, turning, and stopping. Stick to bike paths until you're quite comfortable skating, and when you do head for the open road, always skate with—not against—traffic. Remember: You're responsible for abiding by the same rules motorists do.

As far as technique goes, keep your hands in front of your body at all times, with your elbows in, your forearms straight ahead, and your palms down, as if you're placing your hands on a table. Keep your arms as still as possible; *don't* pump them back and forth as if you're using ski poles, as this may throw off your balance and increase your chances of taking a spill. Travel in a modified squat position, bending at the knees as if you're about to sit down. Keep your weight on your back wheel and push straight off of your heel. Pull your abdominal muscles inward, and don't round your back. Try to stay perfectly balanced on one foot or the other at all times. If you start to lose your balance, crouch lower—don't stand up straighter. If you fall—and you *will* fall—try to stay relaxed and go with it rather than trying to stop yourself with your hands or your chin.

And never, ever skate while holding *anything* in your hands.

Aerobics

The Scoop

Aerobics have come a long way since the seventies when "feel the burn" was in fashion. Now there's a class for everyone. If it makes you sweat and someone can make up a silly name for it, it's now available in a gym or a video store near you.

If you're trying to improve your cardiovascular conditioning and burn calories, make sure you take a class that has at least 15 minutes of nonstop movement involving your larger muscle groups. Some classes, like body sculpting and yoga, don't aim to get you in shape aerobically. Depending on the type of class you take, you'll use virtually every muscle in your body. Calorie burn and stress to your joints also vary from class to class and even from instructor to instructor.

Good Stuff to Know

Look for a class taught by a certified, experienced instructor. Reputable aerobics certifications are offered by the American Council on Exercise (ACE), the American College of Sports Medicine (ACSM), and the American Aerobics Fitness Association (AAFA). You can make an exception for "specialty" classes like box aerobics.

Boxing and other martial arts classes are often taught by ex-boxers who know the fancy footwork but don't teach mainstream aerobic classes, so they don't bother with formal certifications.

The certification rule does apply to video instructors, however. If they have a certification or affiliation, you can bet it will be printed on the cover. Don't be fooled by trademarked titles like "America's Trainer" or "Trainer to the Stars." Often they've been invented to distract you from the lack of real credentials. They are no substitute for valid, recognized certification or education. That goes double for celebrity videos. Sure, it's nice to sweat along with an Academy Award winner (or a has-been underwear model), but sometimes they're not the safest or the best workout. Some of the best celeb videos pair a famous face with a well-known, certified fitness instructor.

Essential Gear

A good pair of aerobic shoes has ankle support and lots of cushioning at the ball of the foot. Most run in the $50 range. You may also feel compelled to spend a fortune on a workout wardrobe, especially if your gym is a scene. But vanity kills your Visa bill. If your gym has a less judgmental environment, be comfortable, be yourself.

The average American spends approximately 25 years sleeping during a lifetime. You burn only one calorie per minute sleeping.

Exercise videos will run you between $10 and $40 apiece, so you can build a reasonably diverse library for around $100. You can buy videos in sporting-goods stores, in record stores, in the supermarket, or through specialty catalogs, or you can rent them from your local video store. As inexpensive as it is to own or rent your own videos, be aware that home aerobics can have hidden costs if they require exercise paraphernalia like exercise rubber bands ($10), a step ($40), a slide trainer ($60), or weights ($100 or more). Dropping this kind of cash, you may feel like you two are dating.

Tips for Rookies

At first, look for classes with the word "beginning," "basic," or "fundamental" in the title; the same applies to exercise videos. Let an instructor know if it's your first time taking a class; he should ask for class virgins before starting the class anyway and also about injuries or limitations like knee, back, or neck problems.

Listen to your body. The instructor may be encouraging you to keep going or you may get caught up by the mood of the class, but if your body says no, let it have the final word. Only do as much as you can and skip any move that doesn't feel right; no need to feel embarrassed if you can't make it all the way through. You can always march in place instead of following along; if you're doing a tape, press the pause button and walk slowly around the room until you're ready for more. Start with two or three 30–60-minute classes a week and build slowly.

Aerobic Machines
The Scoop

Whether you're into mountain climbing,

CALORIES: baked, fried, or roasted?	
Activity	Calories Burned 30 Minutes Slow / Fast
Aerobics	175–270
Box Aerobics	130–180
Cross-Country Skiing	175–360
Cycling	130–210
Jogging (10–12-minute miles)	255–300
Jump Rope	265–340
Rowing	130–230
Running (8–10-minute miles)	330–400
Skating, Lateral Movement Training (slide)	302–380
Stair Climbing	243–288
Step Aerobics	184–225
Swimming (crawl stroke)	130–230
Walking	130–170

cross-country skiing, windsurfing, or whatever—there's a machine that simulates it. Indoor aerobic simulators are the next-best thing to the real thing. And sometimes they're better than the real thing. Take running up stairs at the high school stadium for instance: A good activity for burning calories and working your thighs and butt, but it stresses out your knees something fierce. Switch to a stair-climbing machine and you receive all the benefits minus the wear and tear on your joints.

The most common indoor aerobic machines include stationary bikes, rowers, treadmills, stair climbers, ladder climbers, and cross-country skiers. You'll also see machines that appear to mimic no known natural activity: gadgets that make it seem as if you're walking on air or you're reclining backward and pushing your feet away from you. If you're lucky enough to belong to a diversely equipped gym, keep an open mind and try everything. Of course, you'll definitely like some machines better than others.

Heading to the gym or purchasing an exercise machine for your home may be more convenient if you work out at crazy hours—and safer if you live in an urban area. Still, you may miss the wind whipping through your hair and the scenery whizzing by. If you're bored by the great indoors, save the simulating machines for rainy days.

Good Stuff to Know

Most aerobic simulators are fairly straightforward. If you can pedal an outdoor bike, you can pedal a stationary exercycle. You may want to ask a trainer or someone in the know about all those fancy digital displays and flashing lights aerobic machines possess nowadays. They provide information about your speed, distance, exercise time, and calorie burn—all stuff worth knowing about and recording for future reference.

Essential Gear

It's a good idea to try stuff out at a health club first if you're thinking about purchasing home equipment; that way you can get a feel for the type of machinery you like. Try everything out at the equipment dealer before you buy it, though. Some home equipment just doesn't feel as good as the equipment you find in clubs. Many people opt for the same make and model they use at the gym rather than the scaled-down home version even though it usually costs a lot more. Just make sure it's something you'll use and not something that you'll hang your clothes on. If you don't use it, don't be surprised if you feel like it's mocking you while it watches you walk around naked.

Of course, there's tons of cheap stuff that will give you a more than adequate workout. A jump rope, a step training bench, or a slide trainer will do wonders for you aerobically and all of them cost under $100; in fact, you can buy a jump rope for under $10.

Tips for Rookies

For those who are into an outdoor sport, simulators are great practice for the actual activity and a useful training tool for the off-season. Sure, the treadmill doesn't feel exactly like running on the road but it might be a good place to get your speed work in or practice hill running.

Simulators are also a good place for beginners to learn the ropes. It's a lot easier to master the fundamentals of mountain climbing if you don't have to worry about plunging 40 feet every time you make the tiniest mistake. They're also good for beginners who are trying to find the right activity. Trying everything out at a health club gives you the opportunity to explore your options without investing a ton of money. They also make cross training easier. Think cross training is some-

cross-training smorgasbord

IF YOU . . .	REPLACE WITH ONE OR TWO WORKOUTS A WEEK OF . . .	BECAUSE . . .
jog 3 times a week or more	swimming, water running, or aqua-robics.	Water activities give your body a much needed break from the pounding and impact of jogging.
cycle 3 times a week or more	aerobics, step training, or exercise video.	Aerobic classes tone all those muscles above the hips that don't get much attention when you cycle.
walk 3 times a week or more	tennis, squash, or racquetball.	Racquet sports are fast-paced and "stop and go" rather than slow and steady. You'll rev up your program and give your upper body a workout.
skate 3 times a week or more	cycling or swimming.	Cycling and swimming get you off your feet. They develop your muscles in an up-and-down pattern to complement the side-to-side movement of skating.
swim 3 times a week or more	walking, jogging, or stair-climbing machine.	Earthbound activities will help speed up weight loss.

thing done in church with robes and incense? Keep reading.

Cross Training
The Scoop

For many people, doing the same workout every day is a real bore. In the long term, it's pretty unmotivating to do the same thing workout after workout—as if you don't get enough routine from your daily routine. At least in the gym you're free to mix things up however you damn well please. Those in the know call this cross training.

Cross training keeps you from overdosing on one type of workout. Alternating among several different activities lets you custom-design your workouts and work different muscles on different days so you get a balanced workout. One day you can swim, which ups your endurance without jarring your joints. The next day you can walk to tone your lower body while you burn fat and calories. The day after that, you can hit the stair climber at the gym to get an even higher calorie expenditure and to shape your butt. Even if you don't want to do a different workout every day, one cross-training workout a week may be enough to jump-start your enthusiasm and keep you working out over the long term.

Here's a good cross-training program: 15 minutes of rigorous cookie eating, 30 minutes of TV watching, then cool down with 20 minutes of napping.

Good Stuff to Know

Cross training promotes balanced muscle development and prevents burnout and overuse injuries. There's new evidence that suggests cross training may also improve your body's ability to burn calories and fat more quickly, because your body never adapts to one thing and doesn't have time to develop little, efficient calorie-saving habits.

Cross training may *not* work for you if you're training for a specific event. Let's say you want to run the New York City Marathon in six months. You'll be better prepared if you run as much as you can between now and then. You can always switch to a cross-training program after the marathon and until you begin training for the next one. You may also want to cross-train if you get injured to keep up your aerobic fitness as much as possible; it won't be as good as concentrating on your sport but it's better than starting

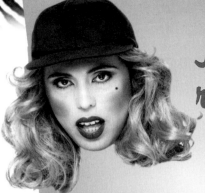

Julie recommends...

7 THINGS TO PRETEND IF YOU GET BORED RUNNING

1. Pretend you're running on the face of someone you hate.
2. Pretend you're running from millions of screaming fans.
3. Pretend you're on your way to the promised land.
4. Pretend you're Speedy Gonzalez.
5. Pretend you're Rocky running up the steps of the Philadelphia Museum.
6. Pretend you're winning the Olympics and stand to make millions doing Nike commercials.
7. Pretend you find running incredibly exciting.

from square one every time you need to lay off.

You can get creative with cross training too. We've described the most popular aerobic activities in this chapter but there are definitely other alternatives. For instance, you could throw in a "stop and go" workout like tennis or volleyball one or two days a week; while these activities aren't strictly aerobic, they will benefit your muscles and cardiovascular system to some extent.

Essential Gear

Obviously, one problem with cross training is it requires the purchase of a sporting-goods store. That can be hard on your pocketbook and take up a lot of valuable closet space. One way to save money is to invest in a pair of cross-training shoes and join a full-service gym. The shoes have a multitude of features designed to protect your joints during many different activities, and the gym should have enough classes of equipment to keep you entertained.

Tips for Rookies

Don't take a random approach to cross training. Choose activities you like that will enhance your fitness level and advance your goals. See the cross-training chart on page 44 for suggestions on cross-training alternatives.

Ready to Get Sweaty?

After reading this chapter you should have a general idea of what type of aerobic exercise you'd like to try (or which least resembles torture). If you decide to cycle and after a few weeks you're hating it, don't let that pollute your view of aerobic exercise altogether. A lot of people hate cycling, especially on the stationary bike. Half an hour of sweating and pedaling is a lot of work to get from point A to point A. A lot of people think they're going to hate swimming and end up loving it. Some people love the camaraderie of a group class while others enjoy the loneliness of long-distance running. A lot of people don't love any of it, but somehow, mixing it up in a cross-training routine makes it suddenly seem fun. If it's not fun . . . if it's not rewarding . . . try something else.

Keep in mind too that continuing to do it will make it easier. People who skate with skill could barely move forward with-out doing a face plant in the beginning. They too were constantly stopping, feeling frustrated. A year later, it's become such a part of their day, they don't think twice about skimming up a hill. It really just takes practice and incorporating it cleverly into your day. The more you do it, the more you'll be addicted to it. Working out in the morning, for many, has become as traditional and normal as fixing coffee, taking a shower, and blaming circumstances beyond your control for being late to work. We promise that, with enough trial and error, you will eventually find an aerobic routine you like, and even look forward to, every day.

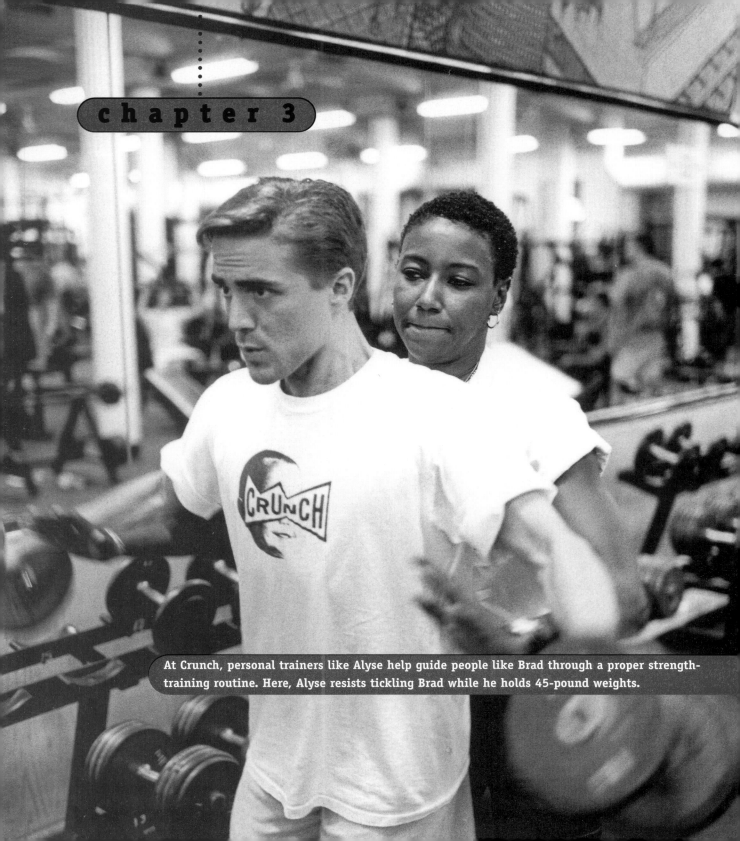

chapter 3

At Crunch, personal trainers like Alyse help guide people like Brad through a proper strength-training routine. Here, Alyse resists tickling Brad while he holds 45-pound weights.

pump!

Strength Training for Weight Control and Toning

Losing Weight Could Make You Fat

You want to lose weight. You go on a diet. You grit your teeth watching your friend suck down french fries, but you do not give in. You do a little jogging here and there, but mostly you deprive yourself of the food you like. You've thought about tossing around a few weights, but hey, you don't want to bulk up and get bigger, you want to be thin. You become grumpy, and even annoying to be around. Sure, after starving yourself for a couple of weeks you see a difference, but eventually you're too weak to jog. So what do you do? You just keep starving yourself.

Two pleasure-deprived months later, those 10 pounds you lost left a gratification-shaped void in your life that you decide to fill with a big Philly cheese steak, cheese fries, some fried cheese on the side, and then some cheesecake. What

the hell! The next thing you know, you've gained back those 10 pounds. Well, now you've blown it, so why bother? You'll never be thin with the world so packed full of delicious cheese snacks. Anyway, you're back to your old weight, which now refuses to pack itself into your old-weight jeans. *What's up with that?*

scared? Studies show that if you feel fearful or edgy, lifting weights can help suppress fears and even help you conquer them. We lifted a lot of weights to write this book.

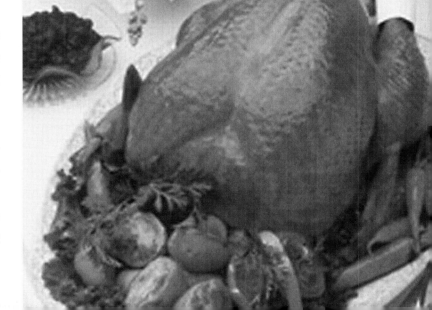

Gobble, Gobble, Gobble. Luckily, a lifetime of turkey-lifting can be battled by weight-lifting.

Well, to be perfectly and hideously blunt, of the 10 pounds you dropped, some was indeed fat but some of it was also muscle or what we call lean muscle mass. The weight you gained back is, as studies show time after time, mostly fat. You don't recover that lean muscle mass as easily as you lose it. Hence, your "fat" jeans don't fit anymore because, although you're no heavier than your old weight, you're definitely fatter.

So a killer body and a dessert menu are mutually exclusive. But it's all right, there's a detour around denial. Fight weight with weights.

From Pear to Bell Pepper

Believe it or not, strength training is the key to long-term, permanent weight management. This may seem counterintuitive if you've always avoided lifting weights because you didn't want to bulk up.

Aerobic exercise helps burn calories and doesn't cause a decline in valuable muscle tissue (like crash dieting does). However, aerobic exercise doesn't do much to increase or maintain lean body tissue either. It revs up your metabolism some, but not as much as it does when you do it in conjunction with a strength-training program.

Add a couple of strength workouts a week to your weight-loss efforts and the bathroom scale will show the same amount of weight loss as you achieved from dieting alone, with one important difference—you'll have gained lean body tissue and preserved your metabolism. In fact, your metabolism may actually speed up. In practical terms, this means your new, lower weight can be maintained with the same number of calories as your old, higher weight—that is, you can eat what you used to and keep your new shape. Now let's go back to that horrendous scenario earlier, where you gained back all of your poundage despite your best efforts . . . that was ugly. But if you included strength training as part of your weight-loss regime, you'll maintain and possibly even improve your muscle-to-fat ratio and your metabolism will remain intact.

Building Strategic Bulges

There are other reasons you should strength-train. Though you can't spot-reduce (that is, selectively zap fat off a specific body part), you can *spot-shape* and, to some extent, redesign your proportions. For instance, working your hips will make them tighter, firmer, and more shapely. Building up your back and shoulders will make your hips appear smaller; your weight may not decrease all

weights

Lifting weights doesn't just make you stronger, it makes your bones stronger. Kind of like an IRA, strength training now helps men and women avoid osteoporosis later, making your life better at retirement.

that much but you'll suddenly look like a perfectly proportioned, V-shaped, firm, lean bell pepper instead of a bottom-heavy, fleshy, soft pear.

Real-Life Reasons to Lift Weights

Lifting weights isn't just a form of narcissism so you can shape up the soft spots and hopefully trim a few pounds. It's also an incredibly smart thing to do healthwise.

People who don't do any sort of strength training lose 30 to 40 percent of their strength by age 65. By age 74, more than one fourth of men and two thirds of women can't lift an object heavier than 10 pounds. This is *not* an inevitability. It's the result of neglect—of experiencing life via your La-Z-Boy recliner and the Home Shopping Network. If you don't use your muscles, they shrivel up and decline in power. This gradual slide can begin as early as your mid-twenties if you're a really dedicated couch potato.

Some good news about all of this: It's easier to maintain strength than keep your skin from wrinkling or your eyesight from fading. People can make significant strength gains well into their nineties. Studies done on seniors show they can at

A reminder from Julie...

DON'T FORGET TO WARM UP BEFORE YOU STRENGTH-TRAIN

Remember from the "Move!" chapter that warming up is important. It gets your muscles warmed up and your blood pumping and gets your body ready for more strenuous activity. March in place, walk briskly, pedal on a stationary bicycle, or play a really fast game of Twister for five minutes before doing any exercises.

least double—if not triple—their muscle power by lifting weights on a regular basis.

Besides sustaining strength, lifting weights also helps keep your bones healthy by preserving bone density. The more weight you can lift, the more stress you can put on your bones; this stress is what stimulates them. If you never tax your bones, they have no incentive to stay strong and dense.

Bone density, by the way, refers to how thick your bones are. Think of strong, dense bones as poles of steel; as you lose density, they become more porous and fragile, like chalk. Roughly 25 million Americans have osteoporosis, a disease of severe bone loss that causes 1.5 million fractures a year, mostly of the back, hip, and wrist. When a bone is extremely weak, you don't even need to fall to break it. Simply bumping into the kitchen table can cause a really fragile bone to snap in two. In addition to fractures, bone loss also can cause extremely poor posture.

Men get osteoporosis less often than women because their bones are denser, but as more men live longer, it will become a widespread problem for them too. At around age 35, most women begin to lose about 0.5 to 1 percent of their bone each year. By lifting weights on a regular basis, you can slow your rate of bone loss significantly—by about 50 percent; if you've already lost a lot of bone, you may even be able to build some of it back. Strength training alone can't stop bone loss—you need sufficient amounts of calcium and vitamin D in your diet too—but it can play a big role.

There's yet another real-life reason to lift weights: It's a good way to prevent injuries. When your muscles are strong, they're also less injury-prone. This may not seem like such a big deal, especially if you're not that active, but if you've ever stepped off a curb and twisted your ankle, you know what we mean. If your ankle muscles were strong, your ankle might not have been wrenched so severely. Strong hip and thigh muscles might have prevented you from taking that misstep in the first place. You'll also reduce the chances of injuring yourself as you get in shape. Runners who weight-train have fewer knee injuries; weight-lifting walkers have fewer ankle injuries.

Muscle Misinformation

Many people have no idea what changes to expect when they begin lifting weights. Or they're afraid to start lifting because they have so many misconceptions. For instance, a lot of people think that once they stop lifting, their newly minted muscle will turn to fat. This is simply not true. Fat and muscle are two distinctly different substances; one does not "turn into" the other. If you stop lifting weights, your muscles will simply "atrophy" (a fancy word for shrink).

A lot of people also don't lift weights because they think it takes forever to get results. Actually, you may be able to lift more weight after just one workout. This isn't because you've built up more muscle; it's mainly because your weight-training skills improve. You improve because, in a way, your muscles have memory. They're smarter than they look. Your nerves, the pathways that link your brain and muscles, learn how to carry information more quickly because they know the way, kind of like how you can get from point A to point B more quickly if you've traveled the route many times already.

After the first six weeks of training, your muscles begin to grow; that is, the size of your muscle fibers increases, you don't actually grow more muscle cells. Most people can increase their strength between 7 and 40 percent after about 10 weeks of training each muscle group twice a week.

Yeah, but how long will it take to *see* some improvements? You'll probably begin to see changes after 6 weeks, but everyone is different. Results vary, depending on your body type, where you're starting from, and the amount of time and effort you devote to lifting weights. In general, those who have the furthest to go make the most dramatic changes.

Also, while working with weights will help shape your body, you'll never see definition—the outline of your muscles underneath your skin—if you have a thick layer of fat covering your muscles. You begin to see a hint of definition when your body fat (the ratio of fat to muscle) dips into the 20

to 22 percent range. You'll be really "ripped," as bodybuilders like to say, when your body fat reaches around 15 percent.

Resistance Training, Not Resisting Training

So now that we've convinced you that strength training isn't just for he-men and she-men and that it's really a good thing, we'll teach you how to do it so you can become a lean hot chili pepper ASAP. First a little background. Then we'll give you play-by-play instructions on the proper way to pump iron.

A muscle will increase in tone, shape, and strength if it is made to resist a weight heavy enough to overload it beyond its normal limits. For this reason, strength training is often referred to as resistance training. Gravity and your body weight may provide enough resistance for some exercises; other movements may require the use of an external resistance such as a dumbbell or an exercise rubber band.

The basic element of resistance training is a repetition, or one complete movement of an exercise. A set is a group of repetitions. For repetition to act as the chisel that will sculpt your body, you'll need to do a small number of repetitions (reps) per set—between eight and fifteen—using reasonably heavy weights.

Do between one and three sets of each exercise. This is high-intensity training and it brings about the biggest gains in muscle and the largest losses in fat.

Get used to the idea of using heavier weights and doing fewer reps; don't worry about waking up one morning looking like the captain of a Russian shotput team. Even people with a genetic predisposition toward muscularity must spend hours a day pumping up to achieve Schwarzeneggerian proportions.

At the end of this chapter you're going to find three different weight-training routines. A routine is a group of exercises that should be done in order for a complete workout—one that exercises all the major muscle groups we'll be talking about shortly. The first routine takes a real meat-and-potatoes, traditional-type approach to weight training; you'll use dumbbells and a weight bench and do basic exercises. The second routine uses exercise bands and tubes and you move from exercise to exercise at a fast pace. It's for those who want their weight lifting on the aerobic side. For the last routine, you'll lift stuff you find around the house, like a bag of frozen corn or a pair of Rollerblades. You can substitute weights or bands if you want to.

One routine isn't better than the other; each just takes a different spin on the art of weight training. It's a good idea to review "Meet Yer Muscles" (below) before any real live weight meets yer muscles. Then go directly to our 12-Step Approach to Strength Training and commit it to memory. Be sure to read the section at the beginning of every weight-training routine too. It's just not weight therapy without a good 12-step program.

Meet Yer Muscles

There are about 650 muscles in your body, and with one exercise per muscle ideally you should be spending 18–22 hours each day in the gym. Not really. There are fifteen or so of what we call "major muscle groups." If you hit each of these a couple of times a week, you'll get a complete strength workout and see definite overall improvements in shape, strength, and tone.

We think it's important to be familiar with your major muscle groups. You know, have a general idea of where each is located, what its job is, and why you should bother devoting an exercise or two to it. If you understand all this, you'll probably get better results from your workout program. You'll know, for instance, which exercises work your biceps muscles, the muscles located in the front of your upper arms.

And knowing where your biceps *are,* you'll realize exactly where you should feel the tension during a biceps exercise.

With many weight-training exercises, it's easy to emphasize the wrong muscle if you don't understand the purpose of the move. If you simply hop on your weight bench and wave your arms around—without knowing which muscle to focus on—you'll be cheating yourself out of a good workout. So let's take a look at those muscles that people will soon be taking a look at. Here's an abbreviated version of everything you ever forgot about anatomy.

Deltoids (Shoulders)

This muscle caps the top of your arm and attaches to the upper part of your chest and to your shoulder blade. Raise your arm out in front of you, move it across your chest, and then swing it in a circle—all that movement is your shoulder's doing. In fact, your shoulder muscle is responsible for just about any move you make with your upper arms.

Strengthening your shoulders can help you avoid injuries like shoulder dislocations or muscle tears. Plus you'll look like you have shoulder pads in everything you wear without having shoulder pads in everything you wear. Sexy shoulders are always in style. Since your shoulders assist your chest and back muscles in many movements, keeping them strong will allow you to strengthen these other muscles more efficiently.

The Rotator Cuff

These are the four small muscles beneath your shoulders; together, they're called your rotator cuff. They help hold your arm in its socket. You use these muscles for throwing, catching, and reaching. It seems everyone has a rotator cuff injury these days, especially baseball pitchers and swimmers, but you don't even need to be active to screw up this muscle group. Something as simple as carrying a briefcase or an overstuffed handbag with a straight arm can damage your rotator cuff. Fortunately any shoulder and/or rotator cuff exercises we teach you will help strengthen this Achilles' heel of your upper body.

Trapezius

You'll often hear this fairly large, kite-shaped muscle located in your upper back referred to as simply the "traps." Your traps enable you to shrug your shoulders when you have no idea what's going on. They also aid the shoulder muscles in lifting your arm out to the side, as if you're signaling the start of a drag race. Toned traps add shape to your shoulders and upper back. Strengthening them may also help alleviate neck and shoulder pain—the kind you might get if you sit at a desk all day, or if your phone is a permanent appendage to your ear. You should give this muscle special attention if you often carry a knapsack or heavy bag over your shoulder.

Latissimus Dorsi (Upper Back)

Not to be out-abbreviated by the traps, this muscle likes to be called the "lats." Small name, big muscle. Actually the largest muscle in your upper body. It runs the entire length of your back from your shoulders to your lower back. You can feel the "wings" of the lats at the widest part of your back just behind your armpit.

Your lats do all of your upper-body pulling movements, like when you open a door, start a power mower, or drag a fallen tree off the road after a twister. Shapely lats help make your hips and waist appear smaller by adding contour and width to your upper body. If you play sports, especially a racquet sport, golf, or hockey, pay special attention to your lats. Runners, walkers, and cyclists also should focus on their lats—and their entire back—to help counteract that tendency toward rounded shoulders.

Pectorals (Chest)

When you hear some learned musclehead talking in the gym refer to his massive "pecs," know that he's discussing his chest. Actually, there are two chest muscles, one called the pectorals major, the other the pectorals minor. Both of them have the job of pushing things around— like that lawn mower you started by using your back muscles, or a shopping cart, or some jerk standing in your way. You also use them when you wrap your arms around something, like five new friends you're giving a group hug after one too many Everclear margaritas.

Strong chest muscles are important for nearly all fitness activities. They also look great in tight shirts. If you're a woman, know that your pecs are located directly underneath your breasts and that by tightening them up, your breasts will appear more youthful.

Biceps

Every time you bend your elbow and bring your hand toward your shoulder you're using the two muscles in the front of your upper arm known as the biceps. Strong biceps make it easier to lift an armload of magazines or carry a bundle of firewood. Your biceps also help out your back muscles when you pull something. Plus, strong biceps make you look pretty buff when you go sleeveless.

Triceps

You'll find your "tri's" in the back of your

upper arm, just opposite your "bi's." Their job is to straighten out your elbow and also help out your chest muscles when you push something. Toning your triceps will help diminish that back-of-the-arm flab that looks so disgusting when it flaps around like a sheet in the wind. Strong triceps will also help decrease the kind of elbow pain you get from carrying a heavy briefcase or from playing too much tennis.

Forearms

There are many muscles located in your forearms which run from the base of your hands to the bottom of your elbows. You exercise these muscles to help prevent and alleviate symptoms of carpal tunnel syndrome (a swelling of the nerve canals in your wrists, fingers, and hands, usually from overdoing something repetitive like typing or playing a musical instrument). It can help with tennis elbow too. Strong wrist muscles will also give you a stronger grip for weight lifting.

Abdominals

The routines in "Pump!" don't include exercises for your abs because we've given them a special chapter all their own called "Guts!" Still, it won't kill you to read about them here too. Your rectus abdominis is the muscle you're referring to when you're talking about your abs. It's the flat sheet of muscle that runs from just under your chest down to a few inches south of your belly button; it's the muscle that controls bending forward from the waist. Your internal and external obliques, also known as your waist, are the muscles that run diagonally down the sides of your rectus abdominis. They handle any twisting or side-bending movements from the waist and help out the rectus with forward bending. Your transverse abdominis runs underneath your rectus; it's there to lend support and stability to your spine.

Lower Back

The erector spinae are the muscles that run the entire length of your spine. They have the job of straightening, or extending, your spine. These are used extensively in Japan when the locals straighten up after courteously bowing to each other. Why bother working them? They are the strength foundation for much of the lifting, bending, and turning we do every day. Many people ignore them, but about 80 percent of adult Americans experience back pain at some point in their lives. Much of this pain is preventable by striking a good balance of abdominal and lower-back strength. Strong lower-back muscles are also very important for getting and maintaining good posture.

Buttocks

We don't have to tell you that your butt

muscle is the largest muscle in your body. Your two buns (left and right cheek) span the entire width of your derriere. They aren't just there for show either. They help you jump, climb stairs and hills, or straighten your leg behind you. You also need your buns to get off the couch so you can go work out. When you do exercises to target your butt, you give it a lift, make it rounder, give it more shape.

Outer Thighs

Also known as the "abductors" by those in the know. These are located at the meatiest part of your hips. They are responsible for sliding your leg out to the side, like when you go in-line skating or do the hokey-pokey. They also rotate your hips outward, like ballerinas do when they stand with their heels together and toes apart.

Inner Thighs

People who know the real names for muscles call these muscles that run from inside your hip to various points along your inner thigh the "adductors." Work these muscles enough and you could squish someone's head like a grape, if, of course, someone's head happened to be between your legs for some reason. The inner thighs are also useful for clamping yourself onto a horse, motorcycle, or mechanical bull. Skating uses the inner thigh muscles, as do soccer and the breaststroke in swimming.

Quadriceps (Frontal Thighs)

The four muscles at the front of your thigh that work together to straighten your knee. You need strong quads for walking, running, climbing, skiing, skating, hopping, skipping, and jumping. And keeping these muscles strong is also the key to preventing—and sometimes eliminating—knee problems.

Hamstrings

The three muscles at the back of your thigh work in opposition to the quads; that is, they bend the knee. They also help out your buttock muscles when you move into a standing position. Injuries to the hamstrings are pretty common. Because your hamstrings are prone to soreness and pulls, make sure they're adequately warmed up before you perform strengthening exercises. Always stretch them after a workout.

Calves

Your calves are the large diamond-shaped muscles that give shape to the backs of your lower legs. The calves spring into action when you need to make yourself really tall to reach the condoms on the top shelf. And strong and shapely calves don't just look good; they also give you staying power when you walk, dance, jump, run, and hop.

The 12-Step Approach to Strength Training

When you pump keep the following principles in mind:

1 Warm up and cool down.

Always warm up and cool down for five to ten minutes before you strength-train. Any rhythmic movement that gets blood pumping into your muscles and prepares your body to work harder is a good warm-up. Any activity that transitions both your mind and your body out of workout mode makes a good cool-down. Marching in place, swinging your arms and lifting your knees to hip level, is the most basic warm-up and cool-down we can suggest. Brisk walking, light jogging, and easy pedaling on a stationary cycle also make excellent warm-up or cool-down activities.

2 Start basic and know what you're doing.

No matter what your level, start out with the most basic version of the exercise described, using little or no resistance until you're completely in touch with how the exercise should feel. Don't just look at the pictures. Read each description carefully so you know what to expect.

3 Follow the routine exactly.

Each routine is set up to start with the largest muscle group and work your muscles in size order till you reach the smallest muscle group. This is so your smaller muscles don't fatigue before you get to the end of your workout. If you decide to pull exercises from different workouts, be sure to adhere to this rule. Work your legs first, upper back and chest next, followed by shoulders, arms, and abs, respectively (see routines for ab exercises on pages 115-123).

4 Do two or three strength-training workouts per week.

Most experts agree you'll need to do two or three workouts a week stressing all your major muscle groups on a consistent basis to reap the rewards of your labor. Major muscle groups include your upper back, chest, shoulders, arms, abs, buttocks, thighs, and calves.

5 Start with one set per exercise if you're a beginner.

Consider yourself a beginner if you've never done any resistance training or have been doing it for less than three months. Beginners should start with one set per exercise. Once you've gotten used to exercising you can gradually increase to three sets per exercise.

6 **Take four seconds per rep.**
Each repetition should take about four seconds to complete: two seconds to lift the weight and two seconds to lower it. *Moving any faster uses momentum rather than muscle power and diminishes the effectiveness and thus the results of the exercise.* Every repetition has a beginning, middle, and end; make sure you move carefully through a full range of motion so you feel every point of the movement.

7 **Lift what's comfortable.**
Over time, your muscles adapt to the resistance placed upon them and you must increase workloads if you want to make further gains. Choose a weight you can lift comfortably and with good form for at least six reps. When you can complete fifteen reps easily, increase the weight the smallest increment possible for the next workout. Your goal should be to use a weight/resistance that challenges your working muscle each and every set. Everyone has different capabilities and starts from a different point, so we can't tell you to lift ten pounds for this exercise or twenty

pounds for that one. You're going to have to experiment to see which weights work best for each exercise.

8 **Exhale when exerting; inhale when releasing.**
Exhale strongly through the mouth during the exertion phase of each exercise and inhale through your nose as you release the effort. Don't get too hung up on this at first. The main thing to remember is not to hold your breath—a common mistake with beginning exercisers. With a little experience, correct breathing patterns will become second nature.

9 **Give muscles 48 hours to recover.**
Always rest a muscle at least 48 hours in between workout sessions. Strength training tears your muscle fibers down; they need time to recover, repair, rebuild. If you want to lift more often than two or three times a week, you can split up your routine by working different muscles on different days.

10 **Rest 90 seconds between sets.**
Between sets, you need to strike a balance between just enough time so your muscles can completely recover

but not so much time that you lose the focus of your workout. When you're first learning an exercise, you'll probably need to take a full 90 seconds of rest between sets, but the fitter you get, the less rest you'll need. Gradually cut your between-set rest periods down to 30 seconds or so. For the circuit training (see Routine 2 beginning on page 76), you'll take between zero and 15 seconds of rest between sets.

11 Don't overdo it.

You want your workouts to cause a minimum of what we call delayed onset of muscle soreness. This is a condition thought to be caused by waste products and fluids flooding into mi-croscopic tears in the muscles. No one knows why this causes soreness 24 to 48 hours after a hard workout, but believe us, it does. If you wake up a day or two after a workout and can't move—begging a friend to hand-feed you—well, you've probably overdone it. If your muscles feel a little achy and stiff after your first few sessions, you've done the right amount of training. Increase the intensity of your workouts slowly to sidestep soreness altogether.

12 Listen to your muscles.

Of course, these are general guidelines. Listen to your body. It'll tell you loud and clear how and when to proceed.

exercises using weights and a step bench

routines

Weight training has that word "routine" in there, but only in the most positive sense of the word. These routines are more closely related to a dance routine or a gymnastic routine than a daily routine, routine emergency, routine fire drill, or routine body-cavity search.

Personality Profile

This routine is for people with the time and patience for equipment like dumbbells and step benches. It's also for people who like that "yes, I'm a weight lifter" feeling of pumping hard, cold steel. Dumbbells and a bench are simple tools of the trade.

Equipment You'll Need

Dumbbells come in all different shapes and sizes. You'll find everything from glitzy chrome "beauty bells" to industrial grays with the hexagonal ends. It really doesn't matter what type of dumbbell you use as long as they're of high quality and in reasonable condition.

You'll need several sets of dumbbells; most people need 6–8 pairs of dumbbells to get an adequate workout. That's because you usually don't use the same weight for each exercise. In general, exercises that work larger muscle groups require more weight and exercises that work smaller muscles require less weight. Makes sense. Choose a weight you can lift comfortably for 8–15 reps. When you can do 15 reps with ease, move up in weight.

You can purchase a bench specially designed for weight training or, as we recommend, a step bench. Step benches are relatively inexpensive (they cost between

$30 and $100). You can also use them for aerobic and stretching activities. Step benches are generally rectangular and come with several sets of framelike contraptions called "risers" you can stick underneath the platform to increase the height. A good bench will also have some rubberized material on top to prevent you from sliding around.

What to Do

If you're a beginner, do one set of 8–15 reps of each exercise in this routine. Remember, do them in the order they're listed so you work your larger muscles before your smaller muscles. Rest about 90 seconds in between each exercise or longer if you need to. Once you feel like you're getting into shape, you can do up to three sets of each. Other ways to challenge yourself: Increase the amount of weight you lift, try out the harder version of the exercise, or cut down the amount of rest you take between sets to as little as 30 seconds.

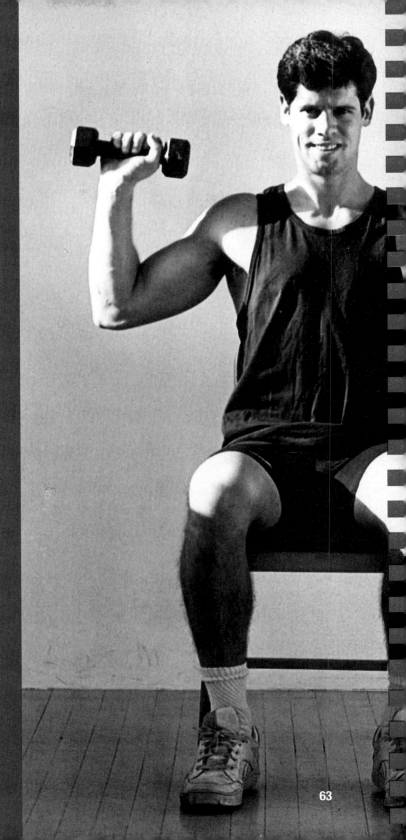

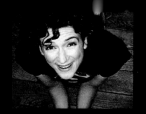

Terry Walsh is outgoing, fun, and loves to show people how to do moves like this one. She is nice but doesn't put up with crap. Do not taunt Terry if you see her. She means business.

Step-up Lunge

A mega-serious butt, thigh, and calf toner!

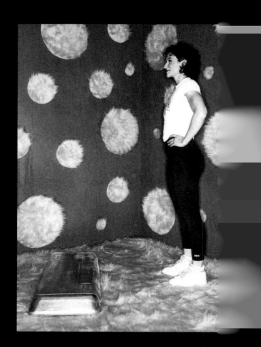

The Setup Place a step (with no risers) lengthwise and about a stride length in front of you. Stand tall behind the center of the step with your feet hip width apart, hands on your hips.

The Move Leading with your heel, step your left foot forward so that your entire foot lands on top of the step. As your foot contacts the step, bend both knees until your left thigh is parallel to the floor and your right thigh is perpendicular to it. (Your right heel will lift up off the floor.) Press off the ball of your foot and spring lightly back to the start. Don't lean forward or allow your working knee to travel forward of your toes. Do an equal number of reps with your right leg.

Thinking with Your Muscles Pretend you're trying to step over a crack in the sidewalk. You'll feel your buttocks and thighs working as you bend your knees and as you push off to return to the start.

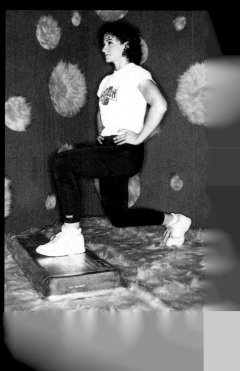

Easier Remove the step and begin with your legs in the straddled position; dip up and down by bending and straightening your knees. (You may hold on to a sturdy chair for support.)

Harder Remove the step. Alternate legs so that you travel forward with each repetition. Swing your arms to help power and balance the move.

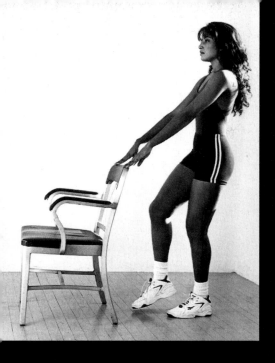
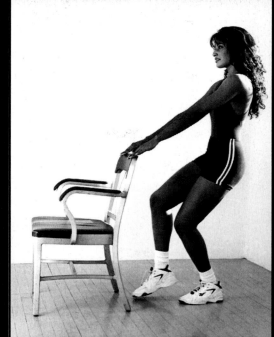

Single-Leg Squats

A fabulous thigh and butt sculptor!

The Setup Stand tall about an arm's length away from a sturdy chair; hold on to it with your hands for support. Extend your right leg a small way in front of you with a slightly bent knee; lift your right heel and inside edge of your foot a small way off the floor. Sit back into your left leg so that most of your weight is supported on it.

The Move While maintaining good posture, bend your left knee about six inches and lower your body a few inches toward the floor; your right leg will remain stationary. As you hold a moment, squeeze your buns together. Return to the start, taking care not to fully lock your knees. Switch legs and do an equal number of repetitions.

Thinking with Your Muscles You're doing this exercise correctly when you feel the muscles in the front of your thigh contracting both on the way up and on the way down.

Easier Bend your knee only about three inches.

Harder Lift your right foot up a few inches off the floor as you lower into the squat position or hold a dumbbell in the hand on the opposite side of your working leg.

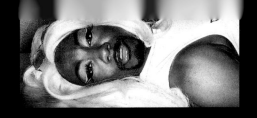

Truly, also known to New York casting directors and agents as Tru Yours, has taught Underground Funk Aerobics at Crunch for five years. Truly often dons a wig and garter belt for his classes because as he puts it, "a subject he's most serious about is having fun, girl."

Plié Slide

A good butt, inner and outer thigh, and calf toner

The Setup Stand tall with your legs about three feet apart, your toes angled slightly outward, your knees directly over your heels, and hands on your hips.

The Move Bend your knees and lower your body straight downward until your thighs are parallel to the floor. Lift your left heel off the floor, point your toe, and straighten your knees while dragging your left toe along the floor inward until it crosses in front of your right foot. Step back out into the starting position and repeat with your right leg.

Thinking with Your Muscles As you pull your leg inward, pretend you're drawing a line in wet sand with your toe. You feel your buttocks and outer thighs working as you step out and lower into the Plié position; as you slide back to the start you'll feel the emphasis in the inner thigh and calf of your working leg.

Easier Do the Plié without the slide.

Harder Drag your toe with more force.

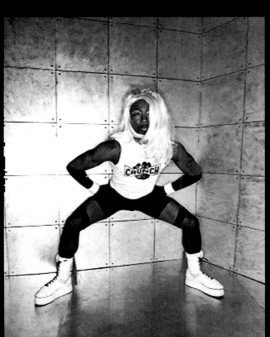

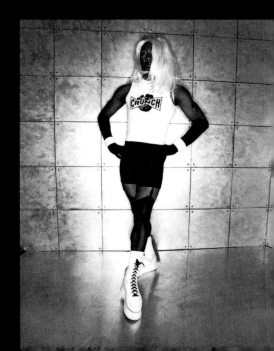

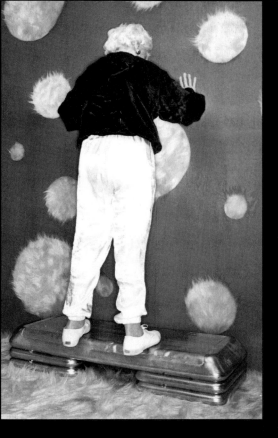

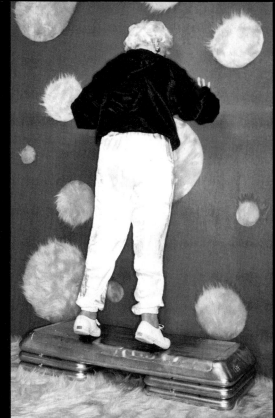

Calf Raises

A grand and glorious calf strengthener!

The Setup Place two sets of risers under your step. Stand tall on the center of the step with one hand resting against a wall or a sturdy object for support. With the balls of your feet securely on the step, allow your heels to hang off the edge.

The Move Raise your heels a few inches above the start. Hold at the top of the movement and then lower your heels.

Thinking with Your Muscles Pretend you're trying to peek over a tall fence.

You'll feel a strong contraction through your calves as you raise up and a stretch as you lower your heels toward the floor.

Easier Work one leg at a time.

Harder At the top of the movement, do ten short pulsing repetitions before lowering your heels. This equals one repetition.

67

One-Arm Row

Works upper back, shoulders, and biceps!

The Setup Step your left leg about three feet forward, lean forward, not by rounding your lower back but by bending from your hips; place your left hand on top of your left thigh for support. Pull your abs inward and keep your entire spine straight. Grasp a dumbbell in your right hand and let your arm hang straight down with your palm facing inward.

The Move Bend your right arm and pull the weight upward to chest level. Lower to the start. Do an equal number of reps with your left arm.

Thinking with Your Muscles Pretend you are sawing through a piece of wood.

Concentrate on pulling with your back muscles rather than just your arm. You'll feel a pull through the front of your arm and the outer edges of your upper back as you pull upward and a stretch through the center of your upper back as you lower the weight.

Easier Pull only half way up.

Harder Hold a weight in each hand and work both sides at the same time.

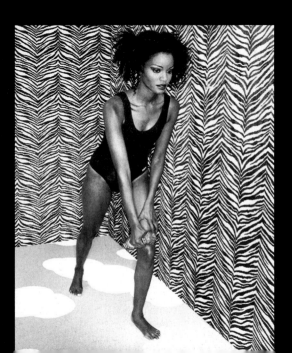

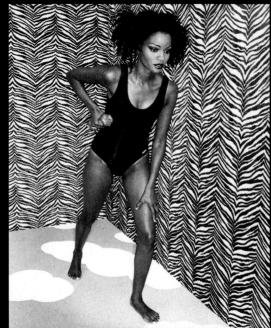

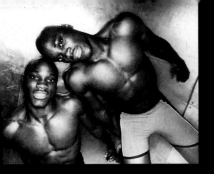

Charlton and Charles are obviously twins. They're also successful models and members of Crunch in Manhattan. They are not naturally bald; this is on purpose. They are adept at strength training and it shows. It is very important to their career to stay in shape.

Push-ups

A killer chest, triceps, shoulder, and abdominal strengthener!

The Setup Lie on your stomach with your legs straight out behind you, feet flexed, toes on the floor. Bend your elbows and place your palms on the floor on either side of your shoulders. Lift yourself off the floor by straightening your arms so that you're balanced on your palms and the undersides of your toes. Hold your abdominal muscles inward and keep your entire spine (including your neck) aligned.

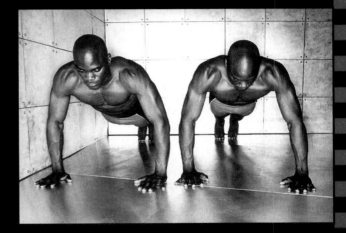

The Move Bend your elbows and lower your body toward the floor in one continuous movement. When your chest contacts the floor, straighten your arms and push back up to the start without fully locking your elbows.

Thinking with Your Muscles Think of your body as a solid, inflexible object that can only move as a single unit. You'll feel a strong pull through your chest and triceps muscles as you push upward. If you hold your abs in tight and keep your back straight, you'll feel your abs working throughout. Women should try this version of the Push-up before doing the easier on-your-knees version. This is easier than you think!

Easier Bend your knees so your lower legs are up off the floor and cross your ankles. When you push upward, you'll be balanced on your knees and palms.

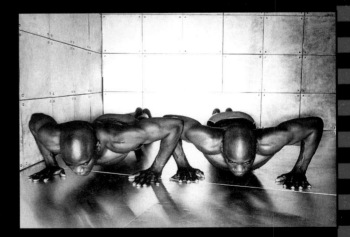

Harder Place your hands directly under your chest, thumbs and index fingers touching.

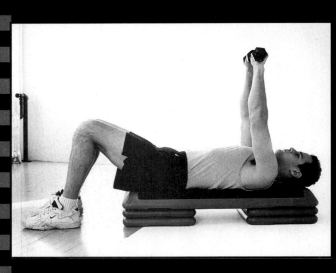

The Se
of risers
high) w
your he
each ha
your sh
and you

The M
elbows
most d
about h
above
of the

Thinkir
tion, ima
a stretc
the wei
as you

Easier
rather
weights

Harder
or place
no riser
head at
you did

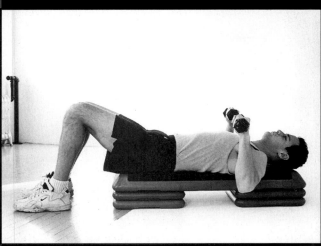

Shoulder Press

Shapes sexy shoulders!

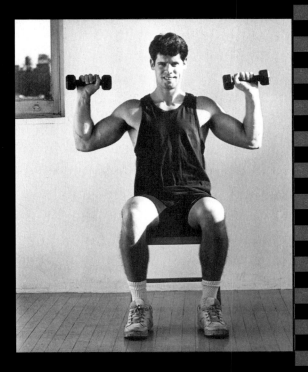

The Setup Sit in a chair with a dumbbell in each hand. Hold the dumbbells up at shoulder height in front of your body with palms facing forward and your elbows pointing straight down toward the floor. Pull your abdominals inward and press firmly into the back support while maintaining a natural arch in your lower back.

The Move Straighten your arms up over your head, gently squeezing your shoulder blades together as you go. Lightly touch the ends of the dumbbells together at the top of the movement. Return to the start.

Thinking with Your Muscles As you're doing this exercise, imagine you're running your hands up and down an invisible wall. You're doing this right if you feel tension in the tops of your shoulders on the upward press.

Easier Alternate one arm at a time. This allows you to give full attention to the form you're using with the weaker arm.

Harder As you lift the weights upward, rotate your palms so that they are facing behind you in the uppermost position. This will bring the back and sides of your shoulder muscles more into play.

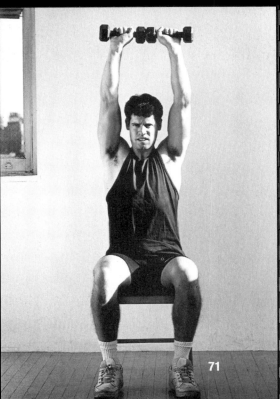

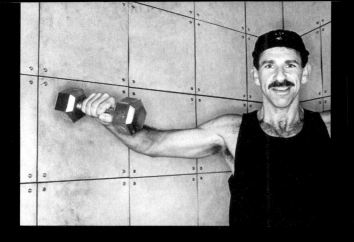

Marc Goodman is a happy-go-lucky, witty guy. He teaches Cuttin' Up aerobics at Crunch, making his students laugh while they sweat. He's been at Crunch for four years. While he may look oddly familiar to you, no, Marc was not a member of the Village People.

Lateral Raises

Tones the sides and tops of your shoulders!

The Setup Stand tall with your knees slightly bent and your feet hip width apart. Grasp a dumbbell in each hand and hold them directly in front of the top of your thighs with your palms facing toward each other and your elbows slightly bent.

The Move Maintaining the slight bend in your elbows, raise the dumbbells up and out to the side until they reach shoulder height. Slowly lower to the starting position.

Thinking with Your Muscles Pretend you are pouring water from two large pitchers as your hands reach the top of the movement. The key to understanding this move is keeping your arms in one position and moving only your shoulders. You'll feel tension in the tops and sides of your shoulders as you lift the weight upward.

Easier Work one arm at a time.

Harder Sit at the end of a step. Start with your arms down at your sides.

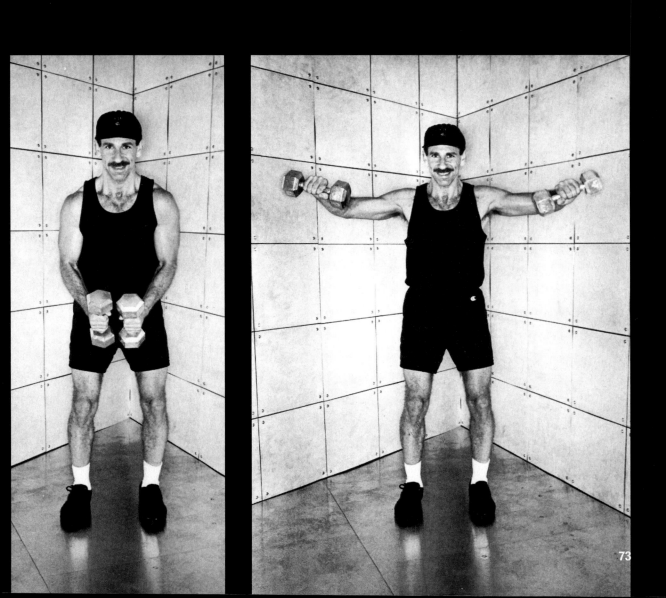

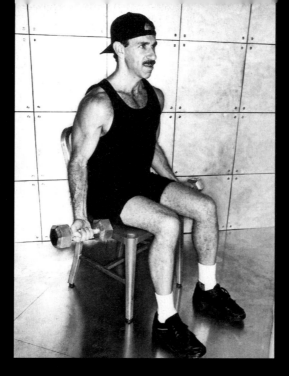 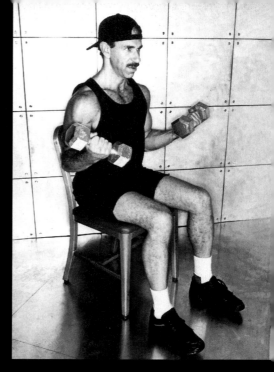

Seated Biceps Curl

A great biceps strengthener and definer!

The Setup Place two sets of risers underneath your step. Sit on the end of your step facing forward with your feet hip/width apart and flat on the floor (or just sit in the nearest chair!). With an underhanded grip and your palms facing forward, hold a dumbbell in each hand. Let your arms hang down naturally at your sides.

The Move Bend both arms at the elbows and lift the weights to shoulder level. Slowly lower to the start.

Thinking with Your Muscles Picture each of your arms as a door hinge slowly opening and closing. You'll feel tension in the front of your upper arms as you lift the weight upward.

Easier Curl one arm at a time, alternating sides for each repetition.

Harder Start with your palms facing inward. As you bend your elbows, rotate your hands so that at the highest point your palms are facing your body. Rotate your hands back to their original position as you lower to the start.

Triceps Kickback

A fab triceps strengthener and toner!

The Setup Stand tall with your legs about hip width apart. Bend forward, not by rounding your back, but by bending forward from your hips. Grasp a dumbbell in your right hand with your palm facing inward and place your left hand on top of your right thigh for support. With your elbow bent, lift your arm up so your elbow rests lightly against the side of your waist.

The Move Straighten your forearm out behind you. Slowly return to the starting position. Do an equal number of repetitions with your left arm.

Thinking with Your Muscles Again, think of your elbow joint as the hinge of a door opening and closing. Keep your shoulder, upper arm, and elbow in place so that only your forearm moves. You'll feel the muscles in the back of your arm working as you straighten your arm.

Easier Lie on the floor or your step and straighten your arm up over your shoulder. Lower the weight toward your ear.

Harder Hold a dumbbell in each hand and work both arms at the same time.

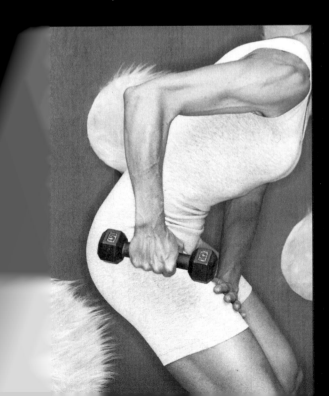
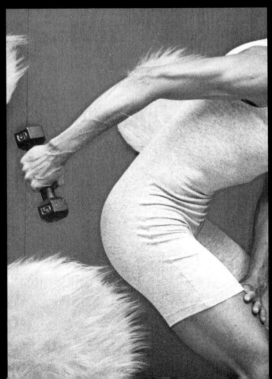

circuit training.
exercises with bands and a step bench

Personality Profile

Circuit training is the perfect training method for someone with an on-the-move, in-a-hurry lifestyle. It involves alternating an aerobic-type interval with a set of strength training without taking a break in between. The purpose: You simultaneously build strength and stamina. Like your life, it's fast-paced and you get to do two things at once.

Equipment You'll Need

You'll need a step bench (see page 77). You'll also need an exercise band, which can be either tube-shaped or wide and flat. Different thicknesses and colors denote different amounts of resistance. They cost next to nothing, usually no more than $10 for a set of three. You can buy them in a sporting goods or an exercise equipment specialty store.

If your band doesn't have handles and a move calls for you to hold an end in each hand, loop them loosely around your hands rather than tightly winding them around your palms. You don't want to cut off the circulation to your hands. Check frequently for holes and tears by holding your band up to a light. If you find any, replace the band immediately to avoid injury and aggravation.

Time your exercise intervals with a stopwatch, a chronograph, or a wall clock with a second hand. It's not easy to check the time during a strength-training interval but here's a good rule of thumb: since each rep takes about 4 seconds to complete, you'll do about 15 repetitions per minute. If you're feeling really ambitious, you may want to make your own circuit tape by dubbing timed bits of music. (Many tape recorders have a feature that allows you to do this fairly easily.) Stick with music that's between 100 and 140 beats per minute. You can also purchase premade circuit tapes.

The idea here is to move quickly from station to station, so arrange your equipment beforehand.

What to Do

Start with the first exercise listed, the

Band Squat, and after you've done 8–15 reps, move on to the first Cardio Move, the Basic Step. Do this for one minute and move on to the next exercise. You'll continue alternating a strength-training exercise with an aerobic interval until you've completed the entire circuit. Once through should take you between 15 and 20 minutes.

If you've never tried circuit training before, start with one-minute Cardio Move aerobic intervals and 8–15 repetitions per weight-training set. For more of a challenge you can increase the Cardio Move intervals to two or three minutes or go through the circuit one or two more times.

We recommend learning each exercise first, before you string them together into a circuit. Because you're moving so fast, there's little time to think; form should be second nature. Note that there's only one version of each exercise. If an exercise is too difficult, do it without the band. If it's too easy, wrap the band tighter or use a thicker band.

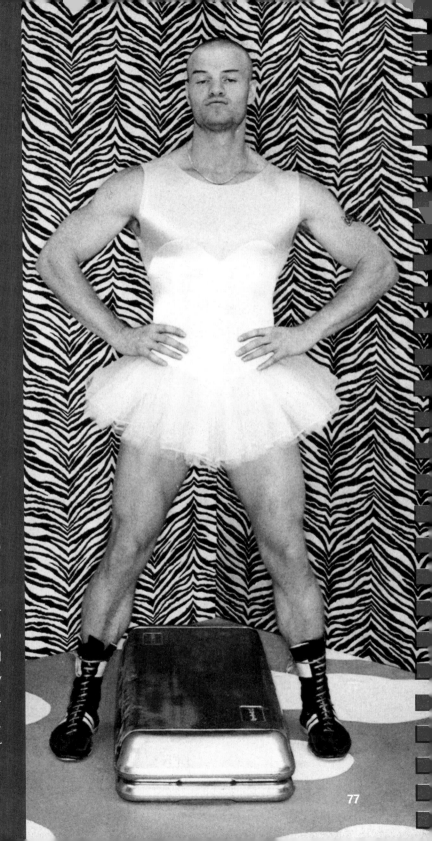

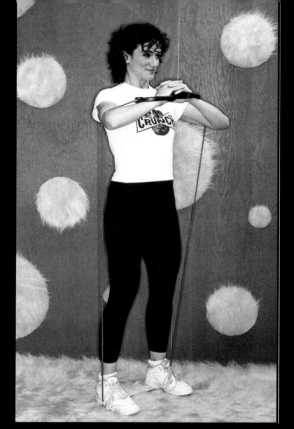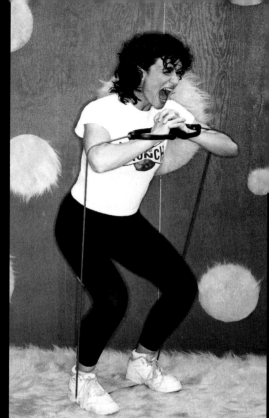

Band Squats

A good butt, hip, and thigh tightener and toner!

The Setup Stand on top of an exercise band, holding an end in each hand. Raise you
hands up in front of your chest so that your elbows are pointing downward and the band
wraps around behind your elbows. Stand tall with your abs pulled in, chest lifted, and
spine aligned.

The Move Bend your knees and lower your body until your thighs are parallel to the
floor. Hold a moment and slowly return to the start, taking care not to lock your knees
at the top of the movement.

Thinking with Your Muscles Pretend you're sitting into a chair and then standing up
out of it. You'll feel your entire lower body working as you stand up, especially with the

No, you're not seeing things. Greg Jones is missing his right arm. He lost it to cancer when he was a little boy. In place of his arm is a beautiful tattoo of an angel's wing. Greg was delighted to demonstrate exercises he uses at Crunch to show that anybody can do them and benefit from them.

Basic Step
Right-Foot Lead

A Cardio Move that builds stamina! Stand tall directly behind the center of the step, arms at your sides. Place your entire right foot up on the step, then your left foot. Return your right foot to the floor, then your left foot. Do single arm curls along with your leg movements.

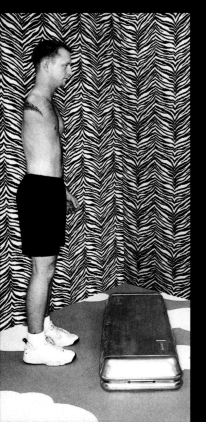
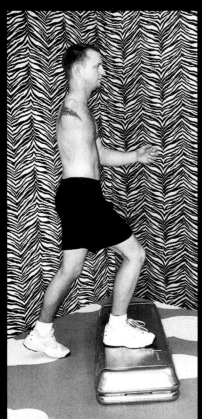
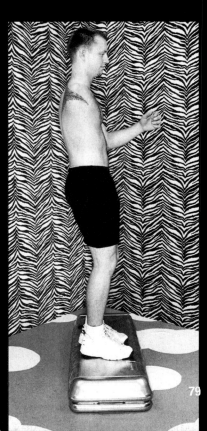

79

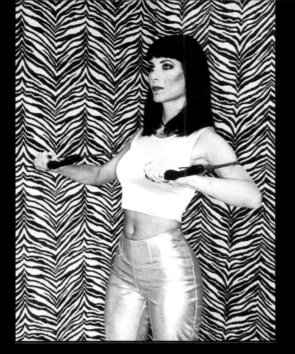 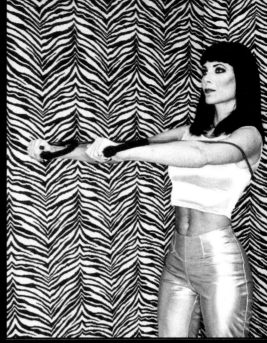

Band Chest Press

A super chest, shoulder, and triceps strengthener!

The Setup Stand tall with your feet hip width apart, knees slightly bent, abs pulled inward, entire spine aligned. Wrap the exercise band around your upper back and over your shoulder blades; hold an end in each hand. Bend your elbows and point them straight backward so that your hands are alongside your chest, palms facing downward, and there is no slack in the band.

The Move Keeping your wrists in line with your forearms, straighten your arms forward until they are straight but your elbows aren't locked. Don't arch your back as you push forward. Hold a moment and return slowly to the start.

Thinking with Your Muscles The band will make you feel as if you're trying to move a piece of heavy furniture. You'll feel a contraction in your chest and triceps as you straighten your arms.

...sic Step
Left–Foot Lead

Same as 1, builds stamina!

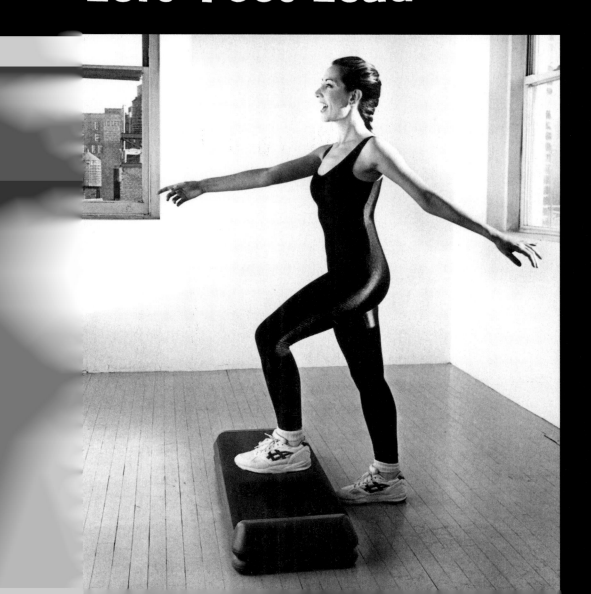

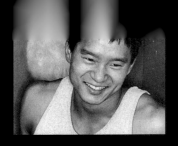

Thomas Kim is a college computer-programming teacher who lives in Brooklyn. He is also a member of Crunch. Thomas uses bands as an alternative to weights. He looks sweet, but is one mean soccer player.

Band Pulldowns

Tones upper back, shoulders, and arms!

The Setup Stand with your feet hip width apart and hold an end of the exercise band in each hand. Raise your arms over your head with your palms facing forward and your elbows bent about three inches.

The Move Keep your right arm still. Bend your left elbow so it travels downward and out to the side and pull the band till your right hand is directly over the top of your right shoulder. In the end position, the band will be tight and your left elbow will point toward the floor. Slowly raise your arm back to the start. Repeat the same movement with your right arm and alternate arms for the duration of the interval.

Thinking with Your Muscles Imagine you're shooting an arrow straight up into the air. You'll feel tension in the outer "wings" of your upper back and the front of your arm as you pull downward.

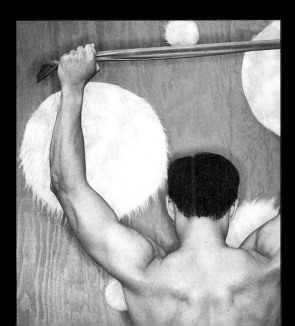
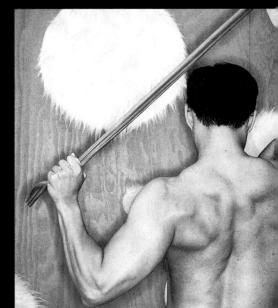

Alternating Knee Raises

A Cardio Move to help you improve your stamina!

Stand tall directly behind the center of the step, arms at your sides. Place your entire left foot on the step, then lift your right foot up off the floor and raise your right knee up to hip height. Lower your right foot back onto the floor, landing toe first, and then return your left foot to the floor. Repeat the movement, this time stepping up with your right foot and raising your left knee. Pump your arms backward and forward to help power the movement. Continue alternating legs.

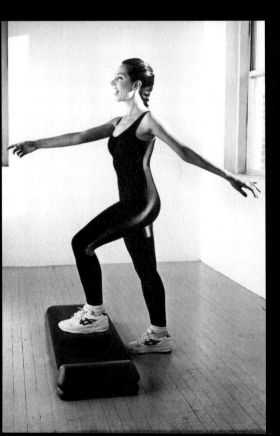
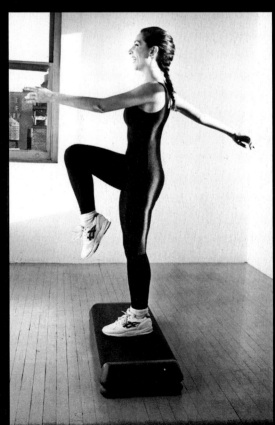

83

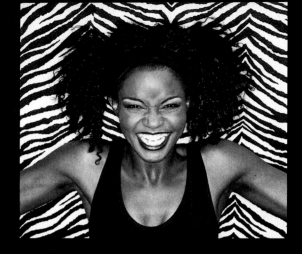

See the "Flesh!" chapter for a profile of Tomiko, fashion model. You'll find her on page 6.

One-Arm Shoulder Press

A great shoulder strengthener!

The Setup Stand tall on top of an exercise band with your feet hip width apart. Place one hand on your hip and hold an end of the band in the other hand with your palm facing forward. Raise the hand holding the band up to shoulder height so that the band wraps around behind your elbow.

The Move Straighten your arm up over your head. Lower to the start. Do an equal number of reps with both arms.

Thinking with Your Muscles Imagine you're running your hand along a wall directly behind you. You'll feel your shoulders working as you lift your arms upward.

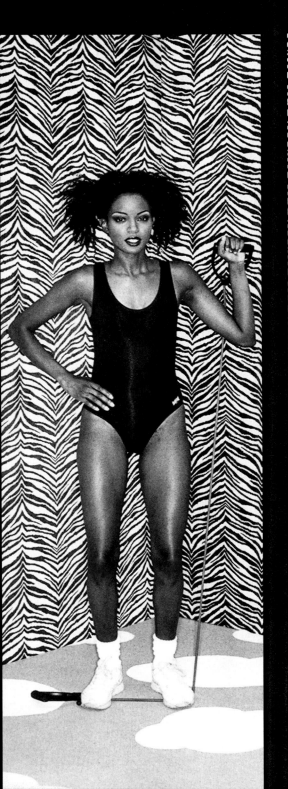
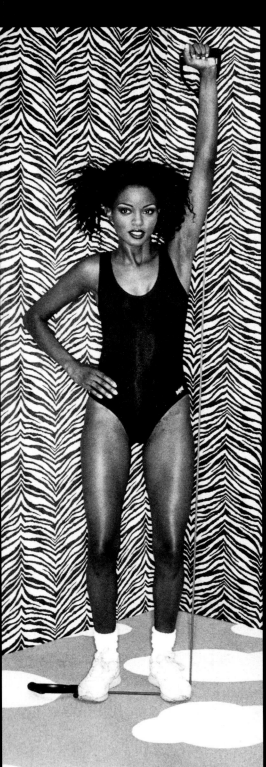

Straddle Down
Right–Foot Lead

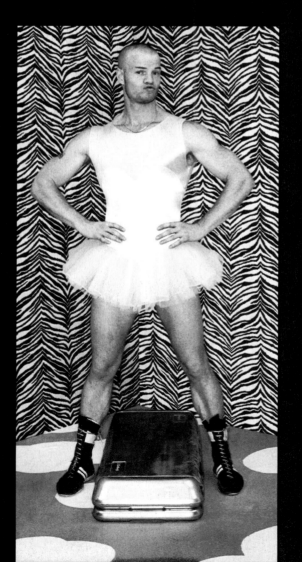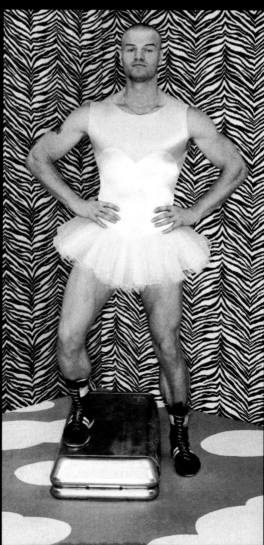

Cardio Move!

Keeps that stamina up! Stand tall facing the end of the step with a leg on either side of the center of the step, arms at your sides. Place your entire right foot on the step, then your left foot. Return your right foot to the floor and then your left. Do single-arm Lateral Raises along with your leg movements to help power the move (or you can just keep your hands on your hips.)

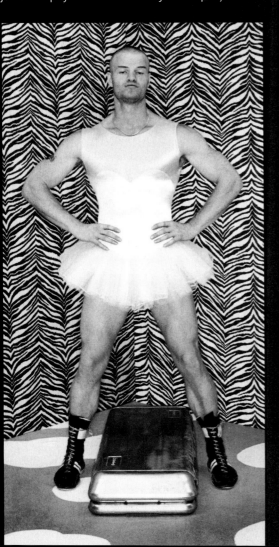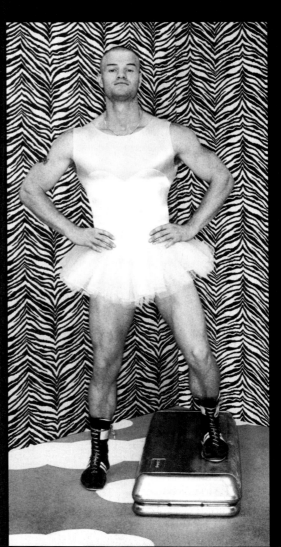

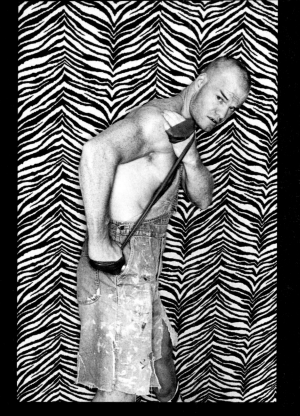
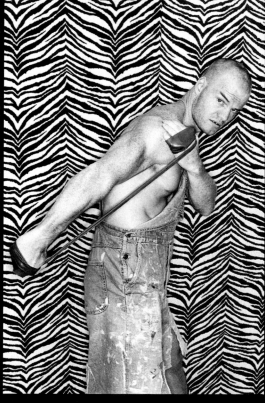

Triceps Extension

A good triceps toner and definer!

The Setup Stand tall with your feet hip width apart. Hold one end of the band with your left hand, then place your left palm over the front of your right shoulder. Hold the other end of the band in your right hand with your palm facing inward. Bend your right elbow and hold it lightly against your side so that your hand is just in front of your waist.

The Move Keeping your wrist in line with your forearm, straighten your right arm out behind you so that the band gets tighter as you go. Don't allow your elbow to fully lock. Return to the start. Do an equal number of repetitions with the left arm.

Thinking with Your Muscles Slowly return your arm to the start so that you keep tension on your muscles in both directions of the movement. You'll feel your triceps working as you straighten your arm.

traddle Down

Left-Foot Lead

to straddle again!

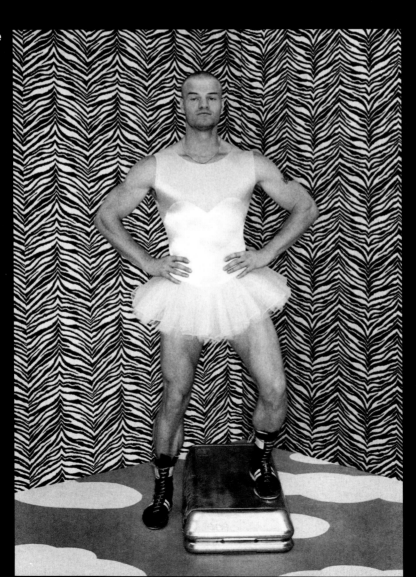

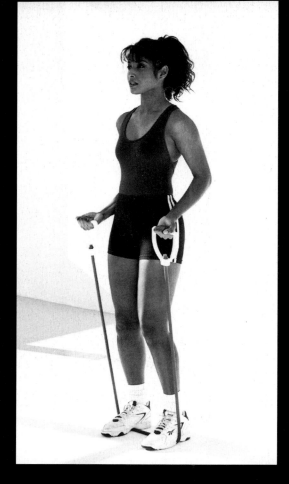
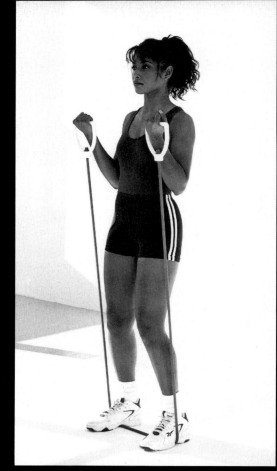

Band Biceps Curls

Builds bodacious biceps!

The Setup Stand tall on the center of an exercise tube or band with your feet hip width apart, abs pulled inward, entire spine aligned. With your arms down at your sides and your palms facing forward, hold an end of the band in each hand.

The Move Bend your elbows and curl both arms upward till your hands are in front of your shoulders. The band will be taut at the top of the movement. Slowly lower to the start.

Thinking with Your Muscles You'll feel your biceps working as you pull upward on the band.

Over the Top and Tap

A Cardio Move for yes, again, stamina!

Stand tall beside the center of the step, right foot nearest the step. Place your entire right foot on the step, then your left. Step down to the other side of the step with your right foot and then tap your left toe down. Return to the start, leading with your left foot. Whew! You're done with the circuit!

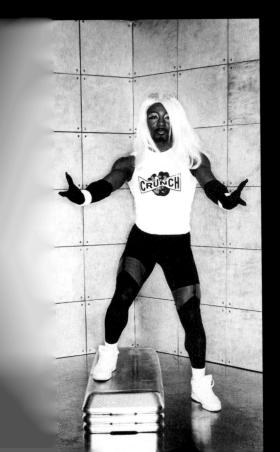
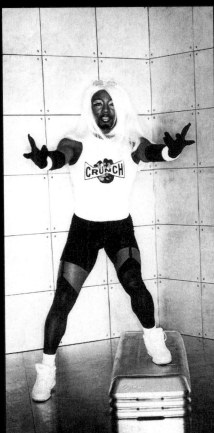
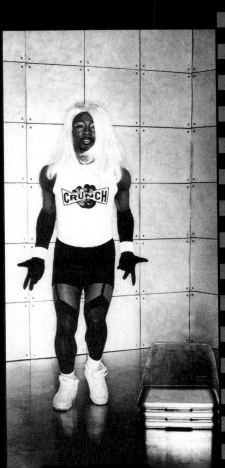

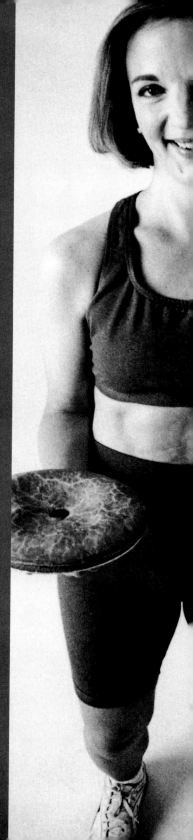

routine 3
no-frills training. exercises using household objects

Personality Profile

For those who like to use what's around the house. Why go through the trouble and expense of purchasing fancy equipment when weight is weight? And why bother with dumbbells when you can improvise? Your muscles can't tell the difference between lifting steel and lifting a one-pound can of coffee beans anyway.

Equipment You'll Need

Get in touch with your inner child by using your Rollerblades as weights. Or lift two bottles of fabric softener while doing laundry. Books, frozen corn, Ajax containers, pies—virtually any weighted article is fair game. However, the objects you lift should be inanimate unless you have a very patient house cat. Weights should be easy to hold with no loose or swinging ends and shouldn't impede the form of the exercise. A can of juice you can't quite get your hand

around or that bends your wrists backward isn't a good choice. If an exercise calls for you to use two weighted objects at the same time, they should be of approximately the same weight, shape, and size. Just remember that the same rules apply to pumping curling irons as to more conventional iron.

Be creative. Rummage through your closets. You were saving those broken table lamps for a reason. Of course, you can even use real dumbbells if you want . . . they're not that complicated.

What to Do

Do an exercise, then rest for a minute or so before moving on to the next one. Though you're using unconventional resistance, you should still do the exercises in order, do 8–15 reps per set and 1–3 sets per exercise. When you're ready for more, find a heavier object. This may present a challenge in and of itself!

Squats

An awesome butt, hip, and leg strengthener and tightener!

The Setup Stand tall with your feet hip width apart, hands on your hips. Pull your abdominals in toward your spine and maintain a natural curve in your spine.

The Move Without leaning forward, sit backward and downward until your thighs are nearly parallel to the floor; don't allow your knees to travel out in front of your toes. Hold for a moment and return to the start by pressing up through your heels. Take care not to lock (fully straighten) your knees at the top of the movement.

Thinking with Your Muscles As you sit into the squat, imagine you're sitting into a chair placed directly behind you. You'll feel the muscles in your buttocks and the front of your thighs contract as you stand up.

Easier Squat down only a quarter of the way. This is also a good variation if a full squat bothers your knees or lower back.

Harder Add resistance by holding two objects of equal weight in each hand with your arms down at your sides.

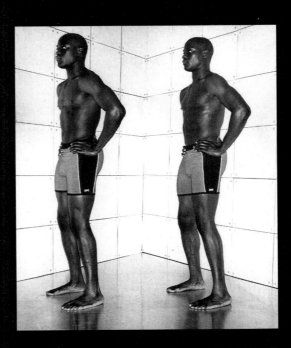

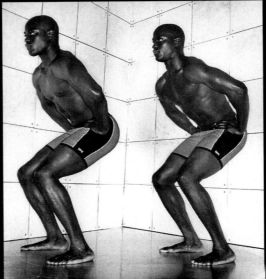

Kneeling Leg Curl

A good hamstring strengthener!

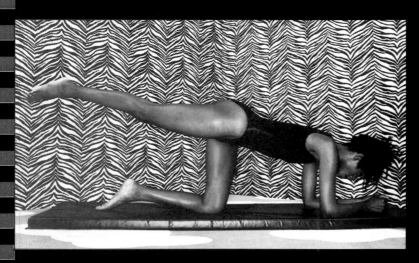

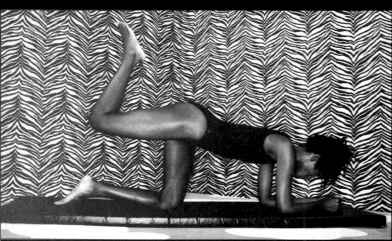

The Setup Get down on the floor on all fours, doggy style. Rest your elbows on the floor. Keep your face parallel with the floor. Straighten one leg and lift it off the floor so that it's level with your hip and flex your foot.

The Move Bend your knee toward your buttocks and then straighten it out again, taking care not to snap your knee. Do an equal number of reps with the other leg.

Thinking with Your Muscles Pretend you're trying to crack a nut with the back of your knee. You'll feel your hamstrings working as you curl your heel toward your butt.

Easier Do the same thing while lying on the floor with your forehead resting on your forearms.

Harder Before restraightening your knee, lower your knee toward the floor, then lift it up again.

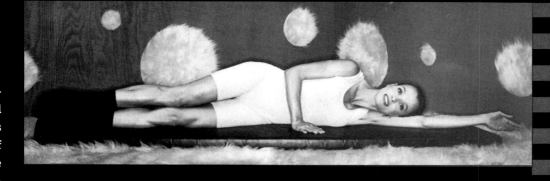

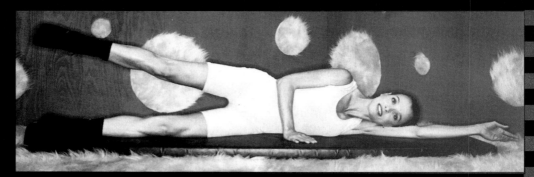

Catherine King is a 41-year-old writer and mother of two. Besides being a member of Crunch, she's a four-time marathoner and a triathlete. She is a supermom and superperson and she's in super shape.

Side-Lying Leg Lift

A nice, easy way to tone your outer thigh and butt!

The Setup Lie on your left side with your head resting on your outstretched arm. Bend your right arm and place your palm on the floor in front of your chest for support. Align your top hip directly over your bottom hip.

The Move Keeping your top knee slightly bent, lift your right leg until your foot reaches shoulder height. Hold a moment and, resisting the movement, lower slowly to the start. Switch sides and repeat an equal number of reps with your left leg.

Thinking with Your Muscles Concentrate on lengthening your leg out of your hip. When you resist the downward movement, pretend you're trying to balance a heavy weight on the side of your leg; that way you'll feel a contraction in your outer thigh both on the way up and on the way down.

Easier Work with your top knee bent at a 90-degree angle.

Harder When you reach the top of the movement, rotate your thigh outward by turning your knee up to the ceiling; rotate back to the original position before lowering your leg for the next repetition.

95

Inner Thigh Lift

Firms that inner thigh!

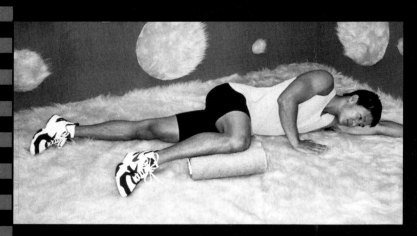

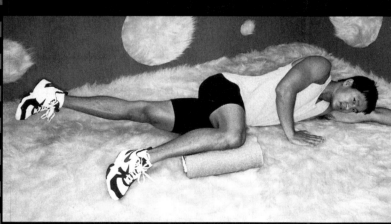

The Setup Roll up a bath towel. Lie on your left side with your head resting on your outstretched arm. Bend your right leg and rest it on top of the rolled towel so that your knee is level with your hip and your top hip is directly over your bottom hip. Rest your right hand on the floor in front of your chest for support and pull your abs in toward your spine.

The Move Lengthen your bottom leg by extending through your heel and lift it as high as you can. Pause briefly at the top of the movement and slowly lower your leg back to the start. Switch sides and do an equal number of reps with the right leg.

Thinking with Your Muscles Imagine a puppet string attached to your ankle pulling your leg upward. You'll feel a strong contraction through the inside of your working leg as you move upward and as you hold at the top.

Easier Place the foot of your top leg behind your working leg.

Harder Hold your top leg up at hip height. Flex both of your feet and angle your toes outward. Lift your bottom heel up to the top heel and tap your heels together ten times before lowering to the floor. This equals one repetition.

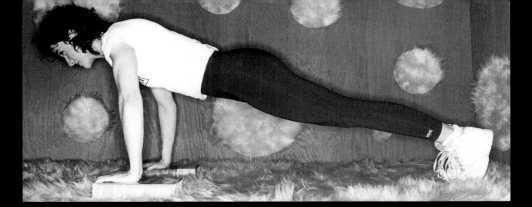

Push Off/Push Up

An excellent chest, shoulder, and triceps strengthener!

tup Place two low platforms (such as
[hard]cover books or blocks of wood) slightly
[less th]an shoulder width apart. Lie on your
[back] in between the platforms with your legs
[stretched] out behind you, feet flexed, toes on the
[floor. Be]nd your elbows and place your palms on
[the edges] of the platforms so they're in line with
[your sho]ulders. Lift your torso and upper body
[off the flo]or by straightening your arms and then
[lift your h]ips and legs off the floor so that you are
[balanced] on your palms and the underside of
[your toe]s. Hold your abdominal muscles inward
[to keep] your entire spine aligned.

[Mo]**ve** Bend your elbows slightly and then
[spring a] small way upward so your hands lift up
[off the p]latforms. Draw your arms toward the
center so your hands land on the floor just inside
the platforms. Bend your elbows and lower your
body toward the floor. As you restraighten your
arms, spring up once again and draw your arms
apart so that your hands land on the platforms.

Thinking with Your Muscles Although we've
described four separate actions to lift off the platform, they should be done as one fluid, continuous movement. (This may take some practice.)
You'll feel your chest, shoulders, and triceps
working in both directions but especially as you
spring back up to the start.

Easier Without springing, step one hand off its
platform at a time.

Harder Raise the height of the platforms.

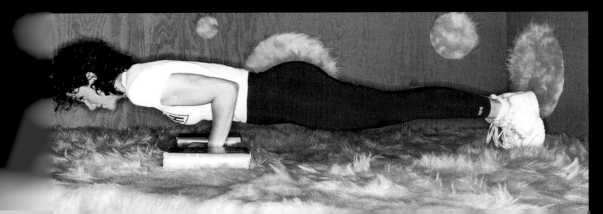

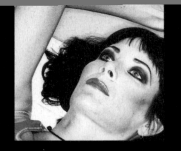

See page 7 to read about Carla Cope (left) and see her perform the Reverse Crunch.

Pillow Pull-overs

Firms upper back, chest, shoulders, arms, and abs!

The Setup Lie on your back so that your head, shoulders, and upper back are propped up on one or two oversized pillows. Bend your knees with your feet hip width apart and flat on the floor. Securely grasp a weighted object in both of your hands and while maintaining a slight bend in your elbow, straighten your arms up over your chest.

The Move Lower the object back behind your head in an arc-like path, bending your arms until you feel a stretch in your rib cage and chest. Hold for a moment at the bottom of the movement for an additional stretch and then lift back to the start, retracing the arc-like path.

Thinking with Your Muscles Thoug your arms are moving, concentrate c powering the weight upward with yo larger, stronger back muscles. If this done correctly, you'll feel a stretch in yo chest, shoulders, and rib cage as th weight moves downward and as you ho at the bottom; you'll feel the upwa movement in your arms and outer "wing of your upper back.

Easier Lie on the floor to restrict yo range of movement.

Harder Immediately follow your last rep etition with a set of chest presses (raisir and lowering the weight directly ov your chest).

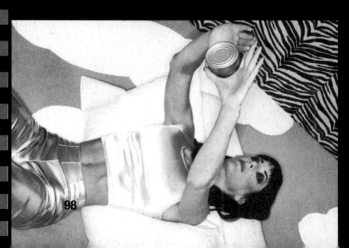

98

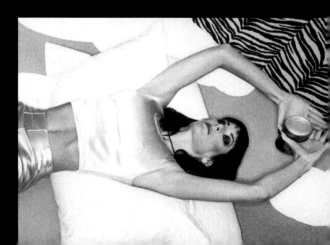

Pillow Incline Flyes

A fab chest toner!

The Setup Lie on your back so that your head, shoulders, and upper back are propped up on one or two oversized pillows. Bend your knees with your feet hip/width apart and flat on the floor. Grasp a weighted object in each hand and straighten your arms up directly over your shoulders so that your elbows are slightly bent, your palms are facing in, and the objects are touching each other.

The Move Slowly lower your arms in a semicircle by bending your elbows and bringing your arms out to the side. In the most downward position your elbows will be bent about halfway and your hands will be a few inches above chest level. Hold for a moment at the bottom of the movement till you feel a stretch through your chest. Return to the start.

Thinking with Your Muscles In the lowered position, imagine you're hugging your Aunt Harriet, who's a bit overweight. You'll feel a stretch through your chest as you lower and hold the weights; you'll feel your chest muscles contract as you raise the weights back up to the start.

Easier Do this lying on the floor to restrict the distance the weights travel.

Harder As you lower the objects, rotate your arms so that your palms face away from you. Rotate them back to the palms-inward position as you return to the start.

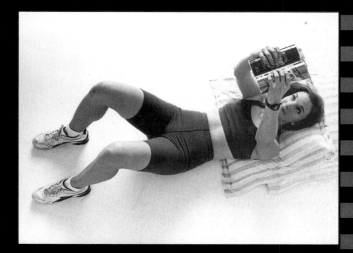

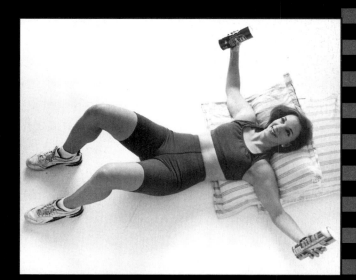

Upright Rows

A righteous shoulder and upper-back shaper!

The Setup Stand with your feet hip width apart. With your hands about an inch apart in front of your thighs and palms facing inward, hold a weighted object in each hand. Keep your elbows and knees slightly bent.

The Move Bend your elbows and lift the objects straight up to your chin. In the finished position your hands will be just underneath your chin and your elbows will point out to the sides and slightly upward. Don't allow your wrists to bend downward. Hold a moment and lower to the start.

Thinking with Your Muscles Have you ever seen old movies of two men pumping the handles of a railroad car? That's exactly what this move looks like! If it is done correctly, you'll feel tension in the middle of your upper back and sides and the backs of your shoulders as you pull upward.

Easier Pull one arm upward at a time, alternating arms and performing an equal number of repetitions with both arms.

Harder Pull one arm at a time, completing all reps on one arm before beginning the exercise with the other arm.

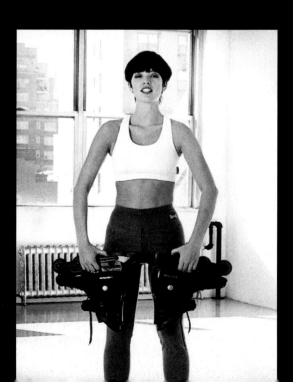

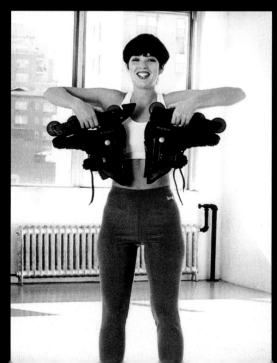

Shoulder Flyes

Strengthens upper back and the middle and back of shoulders!

The Setup Sit on a chair with your feet hip width apart and heels up off the floor. Lean forward from your hips without rounding your back. As always, keep your abs pulled inward and your neck in line with the rest of your spine. Grasp a weighted object in each hand and let your arms hang down so your hands are directly under your knees.

The Move Raise the objects up and to the side till they're level with your shoulders. Gently squeeze your shoulder blades together as you hold a moment at the top of the movement and then slowly return to the start.

Thinking with Your Muscles In the up position, you should look as if you're trying to scoop up a large bundle; you'll feel a contraction in the center of your upper back and in your shoulders. When you lower your arms, you'll feel a stretch across the center of your upper back.

Easier Lift the objects so your elbows travel in a straight line directly upward.

Harder When you reach the top of the movement, rotate your forearms upward until the weighted objects are alongside your ears. Rotate back to the "fly" position before lowering to the start.

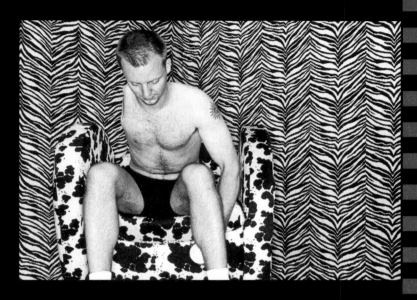

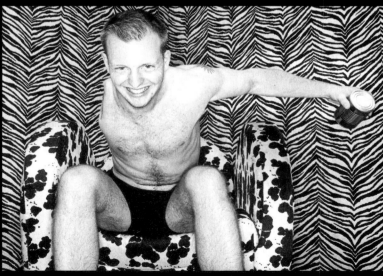

External and Internal Shoulder Rotation

Moves that rotator cuff!

The Setup Stand or sit up tall. Hold an equally weighted object in each hand with your palms flat and facing upward. Bend your elbows to 90 degrees—so that your forearms are parallel to the floor—and press your elbows firmly into your waist so that your hands are together in front of you.

The Move Keeping your elbows pressed into your sides, move your hands in opposite directions away from each other as far as you can. Hold a moment and slowly return to the start.

Thinking with Your Muscles This is a very small movement, so your upper arms should remain stationary. You'll feel a strong pull deep within your shoulder as you move your hands apart; the tension will relax as you return your hands to the start.

Easier Do the exercise without holding anything in your hands.

Harder Do one arm at a time, really concentrating on pressing your arm as far away from your body as possible.

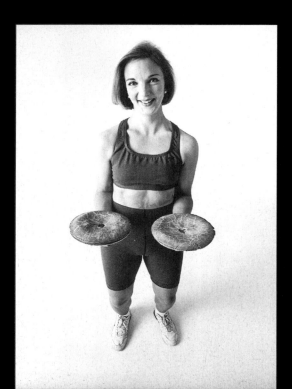 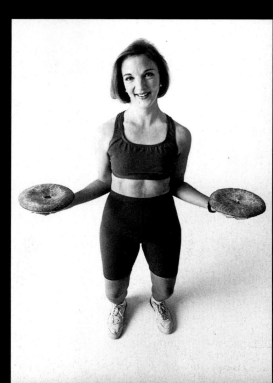

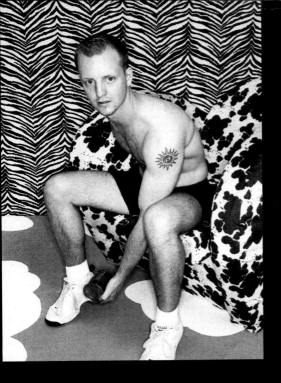
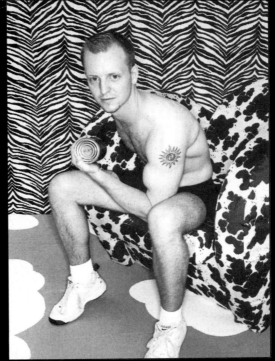

Concentration Curls

Makes your biceps bulge with strength!

The Setup Sit on a chair with your feet hip width apart, heels up off the floor. Lean forward with a straight back and lay your left arm against the side of your inner left thigh just above your knee. Grasp a weighted object and let your arm hang straight down.

The Move Curl the object up to shoulder height by bending your elbow and slowly lower to the start. Repeat an equal number of reps with your right arm.

Thinking with Your Muscles You'll feel the strongest contraction through the cen-

ter of your biceps muscle at the mid-range of the upward phase of the movement.

Easier Use your other hand to assist you through the hardest part of the curl.

Harder Do seven repetitions in which you curl your arm only halfway up, immediately followed by seven repetitions in which you do only the top half of the curling movement and finish off with seven full-range-of-motion repetitions.

Chair Dips

Works triceps, shoulders, and chest . . . firms them up!

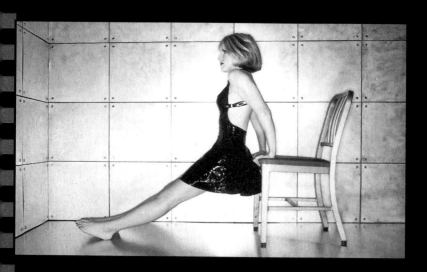

The Setup Sit on the edge of a sturdy chair with your legs together and extended in front of you, toes pointing up off the floor. Keeping your elbows relaxed, straighten your arms, place your hands about six inches apart and firmly grip the edges of the seat. Slide your buttocks just off the front of the chair so that your torso is pointing straight down toward the floor. Keep your abdominals contracted and your spine straight.

The Move Bend your elbows and lower your body in a straight line toward the floor. When your upper arms are parallel to the floor, push yourself back up to the start.

Thinking with Your Muscles Imagine your back is sliding up and down along an imaginary wall. You'll feel your triceps working as you straighten your arms.

Easier Rather than extending your legs out in front of you, bend your knees so you're positioned as if you're sitting in a chair.

Harder Raise your feet up on another chair of equal height.

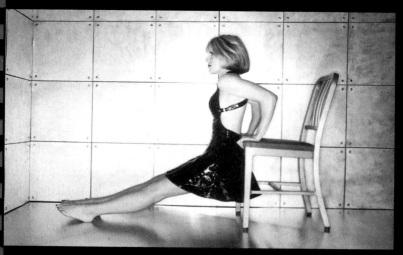

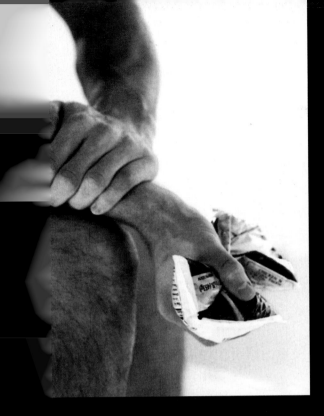

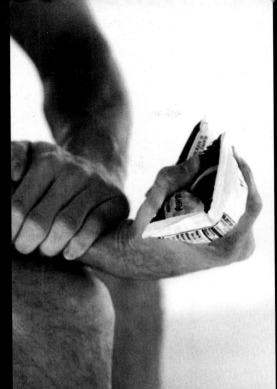

Wrist Curls

The Setup Sit on a chair with your feet flat on the floor, hip width apart. Hold a weighted object in one hand. Lean forward and place the forearm of the arm you are holding the object with, palm up, across your thigh so that your hand just clears your knee. Place your opposite hand securely on your wrist to keep it from moving around.

The Move Bend your wrist so that your hand drops in front of your knee. Hold a moment and then bend your wrist upward so that your hand lifts above knee

level. Do an equal number of reps with the other wrist.

Thinking with Your Muscles You'll feel your forearms get very tight after the first few reps. You'll also feel your wrists loosen up a bit.

Easier Don't bend your arm quite as far on the way up or on the way down.

Harder Turn your wrist around so that your palm is facing downward. Now do the exercise.

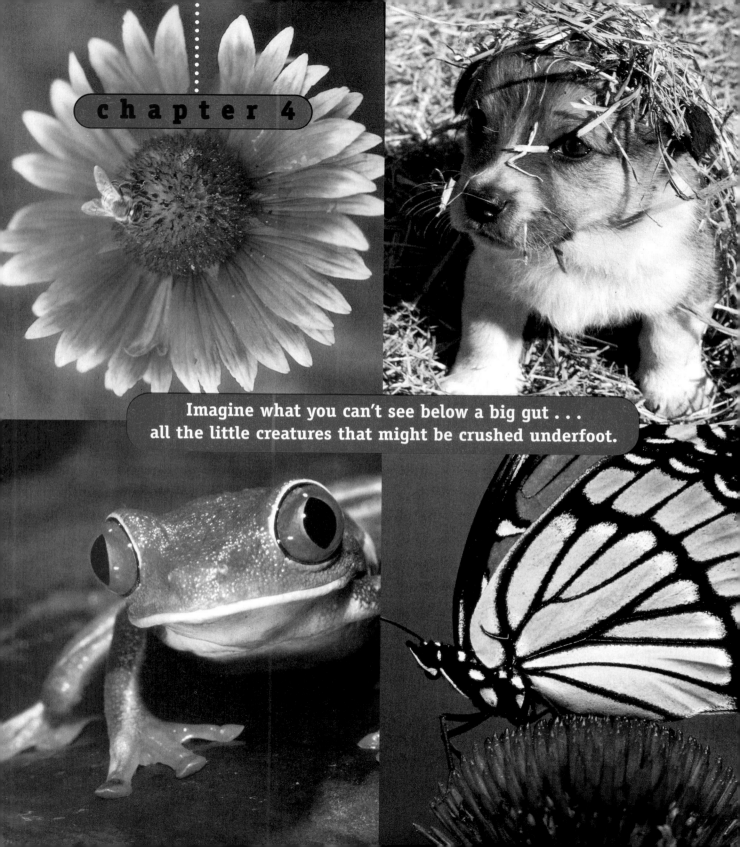

chapter 4

Imagine what you can't see below a big gut . . .
all the little creatures that might be crushed underfoot.

guts!

How to Define and Tone Your Abdominal Muscles

Survival of the Fittest: Why Our Abs Get Flabby

For most of us, a defined muscular midsection seems like the impossible dream. This is a matter of evolution, really. Storing extra fat around the girth is a holdover from our Paleolithic days, when a little extra padding meant the difference between surviving the winter or starving. But here we are in the late twentieth century with magical microwaveable delights and instant meals you sip through a straw. No more hunting down game for dinner in order to store fat for the winter. Frozen burritos don't run very fast, do they? Today, we're not busy trying to survive the winter—we're trying to survive those horrified glances we get when our flabby gut hangs over our swimming britches. Yes, flat, toned Janet Jackson abs (post-1986 Janet, that is) are *the* must-have status symbol in our society. Abominable abdominals are strictly unwelcome. Some of us even spend hours doing abdominal crunches instead of lunches but we still can't turn the spare tire into a steel-belted radial.

Natural Shape: How the Ab Muscles Work Together

The truth? Well, your abdomen is not meant to be pancake flat. It is, in fact, shaped like a cylinder because your abdominal, waist, and lower-back muscles intertwine and work together to form a rounded shape. Women have more tubular torsos than men and are prone to additional rounding, especially when menstruating. Attempting to streamline what nature intended to be curved can be physically damaging and damn frustrating. Besides, there are better reasons than vanity to focus on your central muscles—like strengthening them. A stronger torso does a better job of supporting and stabilizing your body so you're able to stand up

oh, my aching . . . 80 percent of Americans have lower-back pain. Strong abs help reduce back pain and thus annoying whining.

nylon stock up Consumers buy 100,000 Belly Buster girdles each year, and spend 40 million dollars on ab roller gadgets. Gee, that's a lot of belly control.

straight and move with less effort. Ever notice how people who stand up straight and move with grace are more attractive even with extra jelly around the belly? Also, a strong torso can reduce lower-back pain, since the ab muscles help support your spine. Your hurting back keeps you from exercising, but exercising keeps your back from hurting. Follow us. We can show you a way out of this vicious cycle.

3-D Abdominal Training: How to Tone, Define, and Strengthen Abs

While isolation abdominal exercises that specifically focus on your mid belly are the solid foundation of any ab training program, they're only part of the picture.

Think about it. How many situations call for you to bend forward from the waist twenty times in quick succession besides illegal or X-rated ones? No, you're much more likely to use your abdominals (and other central muscles) in practical ways like bracing yourself when you carry a big, heavy box full of $19.95 ab-flab-cadabra gadgets out to the trash. Or reaching way across the couch for the remote. You can't always treat your ab muscles as individual parts or you get only limited results. That's why a lot of ab training programs don't really get you very far, even if you do them diligently.

Complete training includes both isolation exercises and exercises that teach all of your "middle muscles"—that's all of the muscles that attach to your lower spine—how to work together and in sync with each other and the rest of your body. Besides toning and defining your middle, multidimensional training strengthens them for the ways you use them in everyday life.

All About Abs

There are four different abdominal muscle groups and one main lower-back muscle group. Separately and together they perform four different functions. Here's a rundown on everything you need to know about your middle muscles. It may seem like a lot but it really isn't that complicated. Knowing all about them will help you understand why you can't just do the same exercise over and over if you expect to see results.

Flexion

Your *rectus abdominus* is probably the muscle you're referring to whenever you whine about not having a flat stomach. It's the long, flat sheet of muscle that runs from your breastbone to your hipbone and spans the width of your entire midriff. Its main job is to bend your spine, as when you double over with laughter or bend over to pick up a lucky penny on the street; the technical term for this is *forward flexion* of the spine. Pretty fancy, huh? Exercises like the Crunch we mentioned previously are a good way to work the rectus. By the way, there are no "upper" and "lower" abs like a lot of people think. The rectus is a single, continuous sheet of muscle. However, you can emphasize the upper muscle fibers by lying on your back and curling your upper body off the floor (the Crunch) or emphasize the lower fibers by lying on your back and lifting your hips and butt upward (moves like the Reverse Crunch on page 116 do that).

Rotation

The muscles attached to the sides of your

A HANDY LATIN REFRESHER COURSE ON ABS . . .

Transversus Abdominus: The muscle group that only contracts when you put your abs in toward your spine and exhale.

Rectus Abdominus: The long, thin, flat muscle running from just below your breastbone and attaching to your pelvis.

Internal and External Obliques: The muscles that attach to the sides of your torso.

Erector Spinae: Your lower-back muscles.

Novus Ordo Seclorum: Those words under that pyramid with the creepy eyeball on the back of a dollar bill. We think maybe it means "Be careful what you spend this dollar on . . . we're watching you."

torso are called the *internal* and *external obliques.* These two muscle groups work in tandem with each other whenever you twist at the waist or bend to the side. They also work with the rectus during flexion. Firming them up gives your midriff a nice inward taper. You couldn't play Twister, do the Hula-Hoop, or throw a Frisbee without your obliques, but believe us, they're not just fun-and-games muscles: They're connected directly to your spine and play a big role in supporting it, so keeping them strong also helps eliminate lower-back pain. (To isolate your obliques, check out "Twist and Crunch" on page 120.)

Extension

It's easy to forget about the *erector spinae* muscles that run the length of your lower back. You use them whenever you "bend over backward," something experts like to jargonize by calling it "backward extension of the spine." It's not like they're so glamorous or anything; you don't stare at your erector spinae every time you look in the mirror and they don't star in any Coke commercials, but you must exercise them to strike a balance between abdominal and lower-back strength—when one is weak in comparison with the other, you invite all kinds of posture problems and lower-back aches and pains. This chapter has "extension-oriented" exercises on page 118, but you should also read the chapter "Spine!" (starting on page 127) for additional moves, since the abdominal muscles help support your spine.

Be Aware and Stabilize

Exercises that teach awareness and stabilization show you how your abs and lower-back muscles relate to each other and to the rest of your body. For instance, when you move your arms and legs, how do your center muscles adjust to protect your spine from injury and provide maxi- mum power to your movements? Are you conscious of what your ab muscles are doing when you're sitting at your desk staring into space? When you tighten your front muscles, what happens to the back muscles and the side muscles? Awareness and stabilization exercises work all of the abdominal and lower-back muscles we've already mentioned plus the *transversus abdominus,* a muscle group that only contracts when you suck in your gut and then breathe out. Another big consideration for training your midriff muscles to work as a team: Even though your central muscles spring into action whenever you bend, twist, or arch backward, their main function is to work together so you can stand upright with relative comfort and security. If they didn't, you'd be walking around on all fours like other warm-blooded mammals.

abfab
training techniques

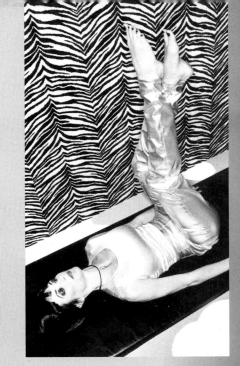

Now it's time to stop reading and get to work on those abs. Before you do this, we want to make sure you're doing things right. You'll need some basic techniques that'll help you get the most from your efforts. Here are some major technique pointers to keep in mind whenever you work your middle:

1 Follow the directions.

Doing the exercises exactly the way we describe them is vital . . . otherwise you may do a lot of work without seeing the changes you're expecting and then you'll blame us for it. For example, we tell you not to lace your fingers together behind your head and not to tug upward on your head and neck with your hands when you do crunch-style exercises. These mistakes can lead to a literal pain in the neck, and they'll diminish the effectiveness of the exercises.

2 Breathing.

Exhale through your mouth as you ex-

ert an effort and inhale through your nose as you release it. For instance, when doing crunches, breathe out through your mouth as you curl upward and breathe in through your nose as you lower to the start. This will remind you to use your abdominals, since more of your abdominal muscle fibers get into the act when you breathe forcefully.

3 Monitor your speed.

Always work slowly and with control. Don't bounce up off the floor between reps or rock wildly up and down to power your moves. You'll know you're moving at the right speed if you feel a

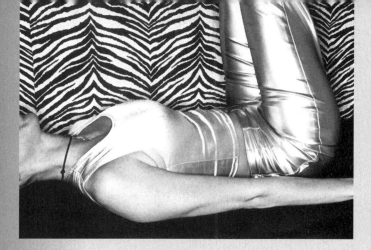

monster baby

The heaviest baby on record weighed 29 pounds at birth. Hope she had strong ab muscles.

uh-huh!

After working out, you should drink water, not soda pop. Sugar makes you lose water, which is why nothing makes you thirsty quite like a pop.

continuous contraction (strong pull) through your muscles both on the way up and on the way down.

4 Anchors aweigh.

Keep your lower back (from just below your shoulder blades to your tailbone) "anchored"—pressed firmly—into the floor during any exercise in which you're lying on your back—unless that exercise specifically calls for lifting your entire back off the floor. This is to protect your lower back from injury and to remind you to engage all of your muscles for the entire duration of each exercise. In fact, the very first stabilization and awareness exercise is called Anchoring and teaches you how to do this.

5 Avoid pain.

If you feel pain in your lower back, your neck, or anywhere else, slow the exercise down and review proper form. If you're pretty sure you're doing the exercise correctly and it still bothers you, *stop immediately.* Try all of the exercises so that you know which ones you can do and which ones you can't. After a few weeks, go back to any exercise that gave you trouble; chances are, your abs, lower back, and everywhere else will have grown strong enough to do all of the exercises pain-free.

6 Don't just go through the motions.

Flopping your body up and down a few dozen times and then declaring "There! I've worked my abs" won't cut it. For the exercises to be really effective, you must focus your attention on the muscles being trained. Each exercise has a section headlined "Thinking with Your Muscles." This is where you learn what you're supposed to be concentrating on, what the exercise is supposed to feel like, and where you're supposed to feel it.

The Rules of the Game

Before you plop yourself down on the floor and start crunching, twisting, and rolling away with a vengeance, hang on a sec. You need to know how to take all of these exercises and put them together in a way that makes sense. How many of each exercise should you do? What order should you do them in? How often should you work your abs? Well, that's what we're trying to tell you:

① Choosing the exercises.

We told you before that the muscles that surround your middle have four major functions. As luck would have it, we've divided our gut exercises into four categories that cover all the bases: *flexion,* or crunch-style, exercises; *rotation,* which refers to any movement that involves bending or twisting your middle from one side to the other; *extension,* which are exercises that involve your lower-back muscles; and *awareness and stabilization* exercises that use all of your abdominal and lower-back muscle groups simultaneously. Do at least one exercise from every category and you'll get a well-balanced, thorough gut workout. We'll tell you how many exercises from each category you need to do based upon what kind of shape your abs are in.

② How long.

A lot of ab exercise programs take up a good part of your day doing what seems like hundreds of sets and thousands of repetitions but you really don't need more than fifteen minutes to get a decent ab workout. As you'll discover, doing more isn't necessarily better; it just takes more time. Beginning gut trainers will find that one set from each group of exercises per workout (4 sets total) is more than enough to start; intermediate gut trainers—those who have been working their middle for one to three months—will need to do two sets from each exercise group per workout (8 sets total); those who are old pros at working out their guts will want to do three sets from each exercise group per workout (12 sets total). It's okay to do a few more from one category than from the others if you really want to fine-tune a particular area, but always include at least one exercise from each group so your middle muscle strength stays balanced. We'll give you a couple of sample routines at the end of the chapter to get you started. When you're feeling a bit more adventurous, you can make up your own.

③ Repetitions.

The number of repetitions we've given you for each exercise is just a suggestion. If you haven't worked your abs in a while, you may find it difficult to complete the minimum number of suggested reps while maintaining good form. That's okay. Start with just one rep if you have to and gradually add reps until you can perform the maximum number suggested. Caution: The most we suggest you do of any one exercise is 20 reps. Doing a few reps slowly, correctly, and precisely is a lot more effective than doing dozens of lightning-fast reps per set as you may have done with other programs. Go for quality rather than volume.

4 When to rest.

Rest between 30 and 90 seconds after each set. This allows your muscles enough time to recover so they can work their hardest when you do the next set but not so long that you lose the intensity and focus of your workout. The stronger you get, the less rest you'll require between sets. (One of the routines we give you, called the Super Circuit Super Ab workout, calls for *no* rest in between sets; it's very challenging.)

5 How often.

Yet another ab misconception is that you need to work your abdominal muscles every day. Nope. Just work them 2–4 times a week on a consistent basis and you're guaranteed a complete abdominal, oblique, and lower-back workout.

6 When to train.

We recommend ab training at the end of a weight-training session or aerobic workout. That's when your center muscles are the warmest and most receptive to exercise. This will also reduce your chance of injury. If you exercise your abs on a day when you're not doing any other type of exercise, you should still warm up for about five minutes with some gentle body movements that loosen up your middle, just to be safe.

And now for the exercises. Here are those great ab and lower-back toners we promised you. Try to keep everything we told you in mind as you go through them. Some of the categories contain more than one exercise; you can do whichever one feels best or you can do a different one each time you work out your abs.

The Basic Crunch

The king of all abdominal exercises!

The Setup Lie on your back with your knees bent and your feet flat on the floor, hip width apart, and a comfortable distance from your buns. Place your hands behind your head so that your thumbs are behind your ears. Don't lace your fingers together. Hold your elbows out wide and tuck your chin slightly toward your chest. Round your lower back into the floor by gently pulling your abdominals in toward your spine and tilting your pelvis upward.

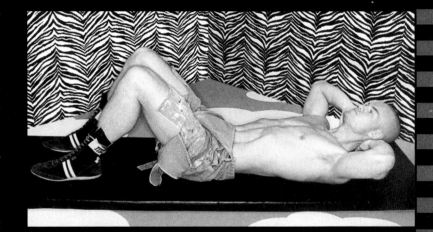

The Move Curl up and forward so that your head, neck, and shoulder blades lift off the floor. Hold for a moment at the top of the movement, then lower slowly to the start. Do 10–20 reps.

Thinking with Your Muscles During the upward phase, imagine someone is firmly pressing on the center of your stomach and you need to tense up your abs in order to resist the pressure. You'll feel tension just below your rib cage as you curl upward; this tension will spread through the entire abdominal area as you near completion of the set.

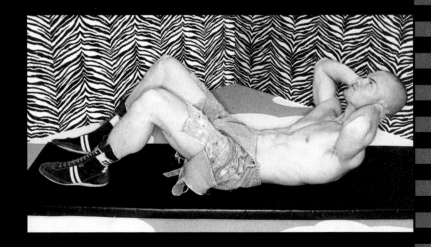

115

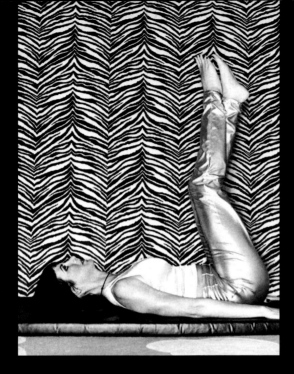
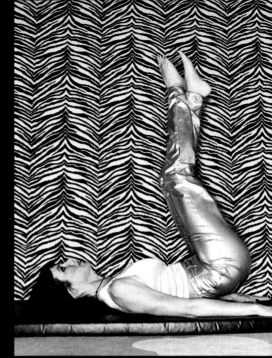

Reverse Crunch

Super-duper rectus ab tightener!

The Setup Lie with your back anchored to the floor and legs off the floor directly over your hips. Cross your ankles and bend your knees slightly. Place your arms straight along your sides, palms downward. Relax your head and shoulders.

The Move Lift your tailbone 1–2 inches off the floor so that your feet move directly upward toward the ceiling. Hold a moment and lower slowly. Do 12–20 reps.

Thinking with Your Muscles This is a very small, very slow, very careful move. Done correctly, there's a minimum of leg movement and you should not allow your hips to rock back toward your upper body—not even a little. That small but precise lift upward will reward you with a strong pull through the lower part of your abs just below the belly button.

Incline Reverse Curl

Gives your lower-abdominal fibers a real lift!

The Setup Place two risers securely underneath one side of your step platform and zero to one riser underneath the other end, so that the platform is at an angle. Lie with your head on the high end of the platform with your back anchored and knees slightly bent, legs off the floor directly over your hips, ankles crossed. Hold on to the lip of the platform on both sides of your head.

The Move Lift your tailbone 1–2 inches upward so that your feet move directly upward toward the ceiling. Hold a moment and lower slowly. Do 12–20 reps.

Thinking with Your Muscles You'll feel this move in exactly the same place as in the Reverse Crunch, only more so. That's because you have to work to overcome the gravity of the incline.

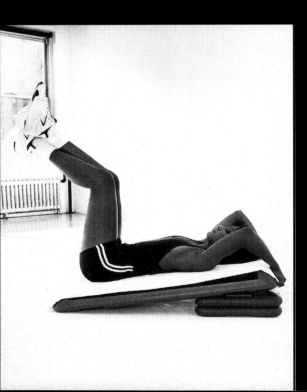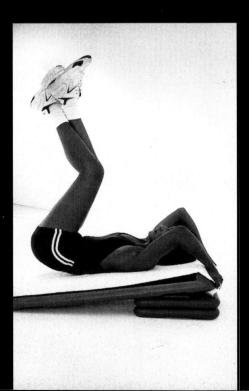

Opposite Extension

Feels good! Helps strengthen, lengthen, and align your erector spinae!

The Setup Lie on your stomach with your abs pulled up and in toward your spine and your hipbones in firm contact with the floor. Bend your right arm and place your forehead on top of your forearm; stretch your left arm out in front of you, directly in line with your shoulder joint, and extend both your legs straight out behind you, directly in line with your hip joints.

The Move Lift your left arm and right leg 1–2 inches off the floor. Hold a moment. Slowly lower to the start and repeat 10–20 times. Do an equal number of reps with the right arm and left leg.

Thinking with Your Muscles Your aim is not to lift your arm and leg as high as you can; rather, it's to lengthen your body as much as possible. Pretend you're trying to reach something with your toes and fingertips that's just out of your reach. You'll feel a gentle pull through your lower back and a nice stretch down the entire length of your body.

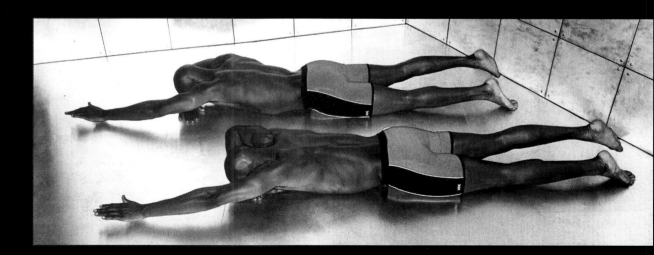

Bridge Stepping

Do it right and tone all those middle muscles!

The Setup Lie on your back with your knees bent, feet flat on the floor, arms at your sides. Lift your buttocks and back up, but leave your shoulder blades in contact with the floor.

The Move Lift your right heel a small way off the floor, put it down again. Then lift your left heel up. Continue, alternating 8–20 times.

Thinking with Your Muscles As you move your feet, keep your abs pulled in and don't let your lower back sink toward the floor. You'll feel all your middle muscles working to accomplish this.

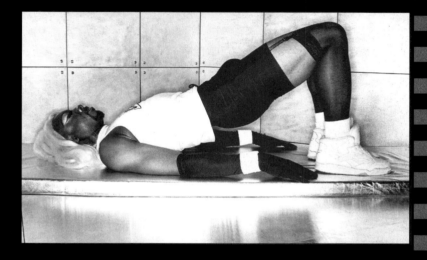

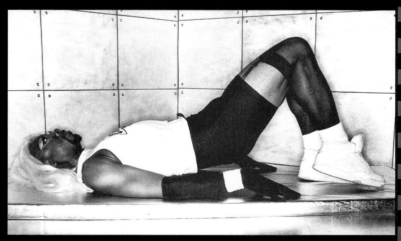

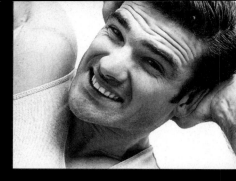

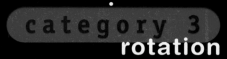

Twist and Crunch

Tones your abs and tightens your obliques!

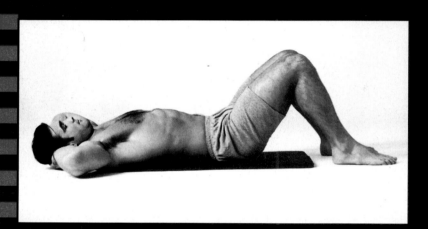

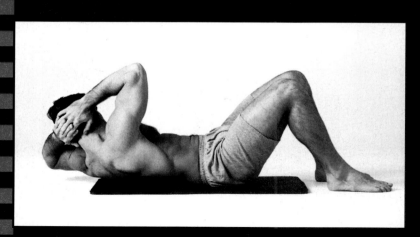

The Setup Lie on your back with your knees bent, feet hip width apart and flat on the floor. Place your hands behind your head so that your thumbs are behind your ears. Hold your elbows out wide and slightly tuck your chin toward your chest. Gently pull your abdominals in toward your spine and tilt your pelvis upward.

The Move Curl your head, neck, and shoulder blades up off the floor and, as you curl upward, move your right shoulder toward your left knee by twisting from your middle (you don't have to touch your elbow to your knee, so don't draw your elbow inward). Hold a moment and lower to the start. For the next rep, move your left shoulder toward your right knee, again twisting from the middle. Continue alternating sides until you have completed 10–20 reps for both sides.

Thinking with Your Muscles As you curl upward and sideways, pretend you are trying to bump something, like a half-open door, out of the way with your shoulder.

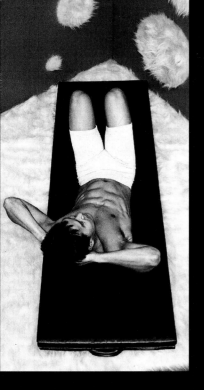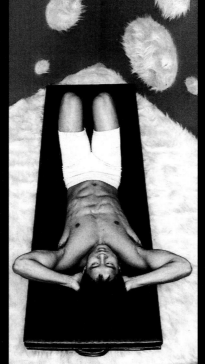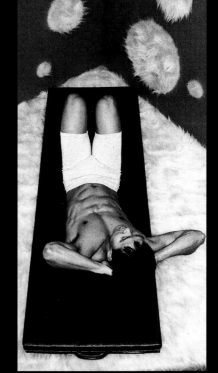

Ab Circles

Terrific waist tightener!

The Setup Lie on your back with your knees bent, feet hip width apart and flat on the floor. Place your hands behind your head so that your thumbs are behind your ears without lacing your fingers together. Round your elbows outward, tuck your chin slightly, and round your lower back into the floor by gently pulling your abdominals in toward your spine.

The Move Lift your head, neck, and shoulder blades off the floor. Hold at the top of the movement. Make a small clockwise circle with your waist: bend a small distance to the right, then lower a small distance down. This is one repetition. Do 10–20 continuous circles, then lower to the start. Do an equal number of reps in a counterclockwise direction.

Thinking with Your Muscles Done correctly, this movement resembles the fluid circles of a belly dancer. Each small, precise circle should trace the orbit of the previous circle.

awareness and stabilization

Liz Heinlein is a very busy TV producer and a loyal member of Crunch in New York. Strength-training exercises help her relieve job stress. They also make her more confident when she dances in her vinyl bra at New York's alternative dance clubs.

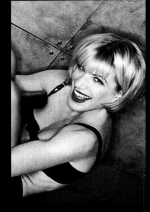

Anchoring

A good all-around midriff toner!

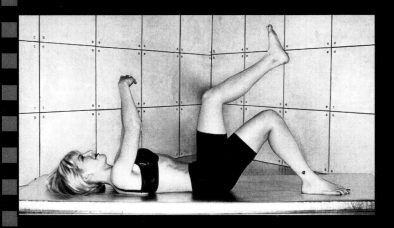

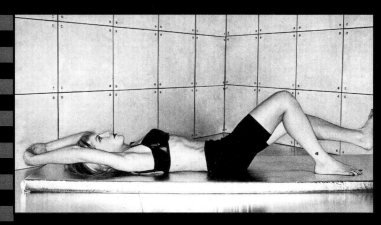

The Setup Lie on your back with your right knee bent, foot flat on the floor, and left leg raised up directly over your hip, knee slightly bent, heel flexed. Straighten your arms up over your chest and clasp your fingers together. Pull your abs downward and anchor your entire spine to the floor. Tilt your pelvis upward by gently squeezing your buttocks.

The Move Slowly lower your left heel toward the floor and your arms behind your head. As you do so, maintain your ab and back anchor. The closer your leg and arms get to the floor, the harder this will be. Touch your heel lightly to the floor and slowly return to the start. Do 3–8 reps with each leg.

Thinking with Your Muscles Being anchored means the entire length of your back is firmly pinned to the floor while still maintaining the natural curve of your lower back. Only lower your leg to the point where you can still keep your lower back anchored. If you can't lower it all the way, don't sweat. You'll gradually work up to it. You'll feel this exercise in your abs.

Double Crunch

Tones and tightens your entire middle!

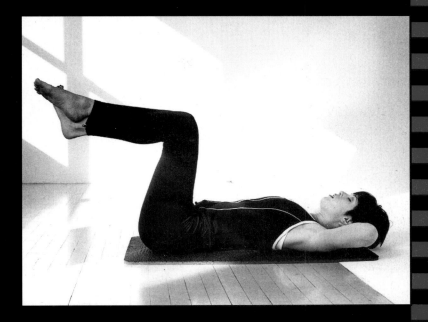

The Setup Lie on your back with your hands behind your head, fingertips touching, thumbs behind your ears. Bend your knees and lift your legs up so that your knees are directly over your hips and your lower legs are parallel to the floor. Cross your ankles. Pull your abs inward and press your back into the floor.

The Move Curl your head, neck, and shoulders up off the floor as you simultaneously lift your hips slightly off the floor so that your knees move a few inches in toward your middle. Hold a moment at the top of the movement and slowly lower to the start. Do 10–20 reps.

Thinking with Your Muscles Imagine your stomach as a bedsheet and you are trying to fold it so that the four corners meet in the middle.

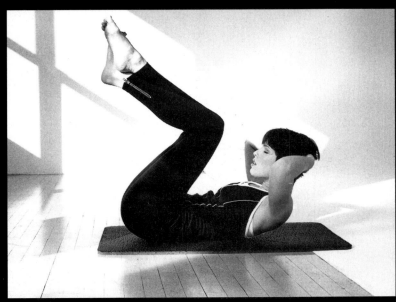

routines

a basic routine for beginners

Including a rest of 90 seconds between each set,
this routine will take you about 7 minutes.

exercise	rep range	number of sets
Basic Crunch	10–20	1
Opposite Extension	10–20 each side	1
Twist and Crunch	10–20 each side	1
Anchoring	3–8 each leg	1

a basic routine for intermediates

Including a rest of 60 seconds between each set,
this routine will take you about 13 minutes.

exercise	rep range	number of sets
Basic Crunch	10–20	1
Reverse Crunch	10–20	1
Opposite Extension	10–20 each side	1
Bridge Stepping	10–20	1
Twist and Crunch	10–20 each side	1
Ab Circles	10–20 each direction	1
Anchoring	3–8 each leg	1
Double Crunch	10–20	1

a basic routine for advanced gut trainers

Including a rest of 30 seconds between each set,
this routine will take you about 15 minutes.

exercise	rep range	number of sets
Basic Crunch	10–20	2
Incline Reverse Curl	10–20	1
Opposite Extension	10–20 each side	1
Bridge Stepping	10–20	2
Twist and Crunch	10–20 each side	2
Ab Circles	10–20 each direction	1
Anchoring	3–8 each leg	2
Double Crunch	10–20	1

a super circuit super ab routine

When you really want to zap your abs, do all of these exercises with
no rest in between. Rest 90 seconds and repeat the sequence 2–3
times. One round should take you about 5 minutes.

exercise	rep range	number of sets
Basic Crunch	10–20	1
Reverse Crunch	10–20	1
Twist and Crunch	10–20 each side	1
Ab Circles	10–20 each direction	1
Double Crunch	10–20	1
Bridge Stepping	10–20	1

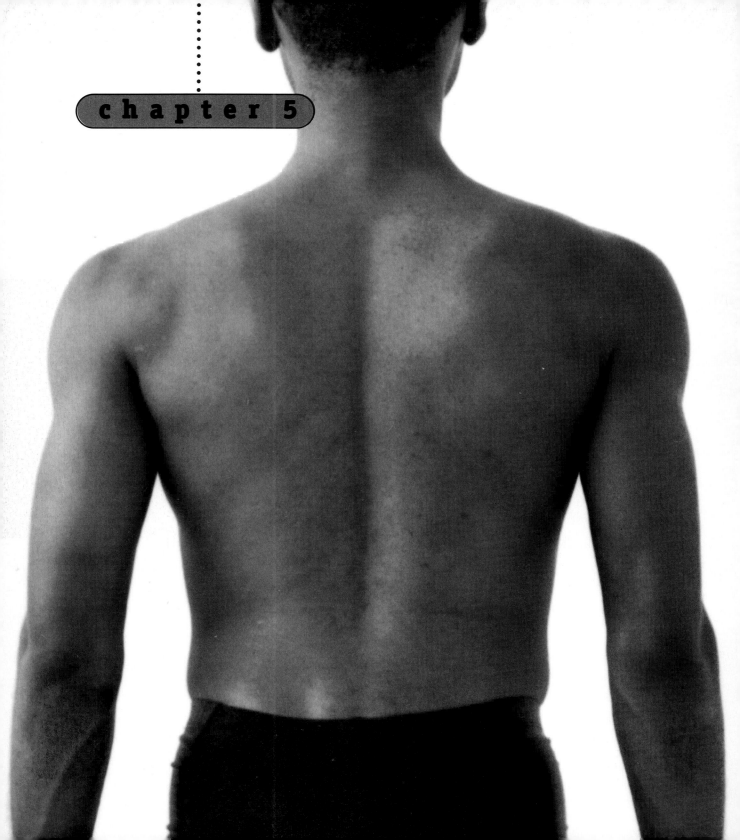

spine!

Strengthening Your Spine for Good Posture and Well-being

Moving Right by Moving Upright

What we normally refer to as "posture" is really a relationship between various parts of the body. Posture is the way you carry yourself, whether you're standing, sitting, lying down, running, walking on your hands, or making unauthorized personal long-distance calls from work.

Considering that most of us have such poor posture, it's a miracle we can stand on the three-hinged stilts we refer to as legs—and even more of a miracle we achieve the feat of upright locomotion without falling flat on our faces! If you think of your body as a stack of Lego building blocks, you'll understand what we mean.

When a pile of blocks is balanced and aligned, all is well. But when even one is slightly out of place, the whole stack is less secure. Well, your spine is a stack of 24 individual bones called vertebrae. It has three distinct curves and runs the length of your torso, starting at the base of your neck and ending at your tailbone. If you think of your vertebrae as Lego blocks, it's easy to see that when one is off, your posture doesn't quite add up.

Say one of the vertebrae in your lower back is slightly misaligned, a common enough occurrence. It'll cause plenty of problems when you're sitting or standing. Maybe your back will feel a little tight, or you'll fatigue quickly. Perhaps you'll hold one of your legs at a slightly funny angle in an unconscious effort to re-align your body—which, by the way, will only perpetuate poor posture.

You'll have more problems still when you decide it's time to move. An off-kilter spine, even when you move slowly, can result in a major pain in the neck. Or back.

> Say you're waiting tables and have to carry a tall stack of plates and don't want to drop them, because that's really embarrassing. Would you rather carry the plates that were placed one on top of the other or the ones that were haphazardly stacked into a wobbly pile? Those plates are your spine and that's the idea behind good posture.

Or hip. Or knee. And the problem only magnifies when you try something fancy like fast walking, running, a step class, riding a bike, or belly dancing. (Although we hear belly dancing is a really good way to loosen up your spine.)

So the upshot of all this? You may be in top-notch aerobic condition or an Olympic-caliber weight lifter but if your Lego set is misaligned, sooner or later something's gotta give.

What Posture Says About You

Poor posture, besides making you feel physically bad, presents an image that is not in keeping with how you want the world to see you. Think about someone you know who hunches over a lot. Does he seem weak and fragile to you? Do you sometimes think she's feeling sick when she's feeling just fine? Do you think he's bored by what's going on around him? Until you knew her, did she appear a little self-conscious or unhappy? People who slump a lot give an impression to others that may not reflect who they are inside at all.

Now think about someone you know with really good posture. She appears strong and confident. He looks like he's paying attention. She's more magnetic and interesting to be around. Frankly, he's more attractive. Maybe the friend who slumps was closer to the front of the line when looks were being handed out than the friend who walks around straight up and square-shouldered. But the attraction gap between the two is narrowed simply because of the way the girlfriend with the good posture carries herself.

Now think about how you carry yourself. Ask a friend to give you an honest evaluation of your posture. It's hard to know all by yourself.

Life and Posture

Though you were probably born with a suitably aligned set of vertebrae, there was trouble as far back as kidhood. Remember your mom barking in front of relatives, "Sit up straight!" Whining in department stores, "Stand up straight." Your dad chiming in at the dinner table, "Your posture's terrible." So what went wrong? Perhaps to fix things we need a sort of psychoanalysis of the spine . . .

Let's take a field trip back in time and pay your inner child a visit. Think back . . .

You probably spent six hours or so a day scrunched into a little wooden desk in class copying off your best friend's paper. Or, if you were the kid that always wrecked the curve for the rest of us (thanks again), think of the posture you had to take to shield your paper. Either way, the seeds for lousy posture were being sown.

Maybe in the third grade you fell out of a tree and broke your leg. Though it healed in a matter of weeks, you continued to walk a little funny. Or in the seventh grade you dislocated your shoulder playing kickball. In the eleventh grade, that's you falling down a flight of steps. All these accidents add up to little adjustments in the way you carry yourself, adjustments usually not for the better. Events don't even have to be this traumatic to take their toll. Maybe you just sat too close to the TV and developed the neck-crunching habit of tilting your head back.

Now, here's the ironic part: Whatever type of posture you have is often partly a mirror reflection of your parents' posture. You've unconsciously imitated your parents' less than ideal stance, like the way your dad slumps in his chair to read the paper or the way your mom slouches when she's worried. So here your parents have been griping at you your whole life about your posture, and they've been partially responsible all along. We'd have a good laugh over this if bad posture was funny. It's not. People who accidentally fart when they try to hold in a sneeze are funny. Bad posture isn't.

. . . You got older. Now you're a fully grown creature spending hours stressing out over a computer or some such grown-up career contraption. Add to this a postpubescent lifetime of spills, trips, stumbles, crazy dance moves, standing in the DMV line, weight gain, that weird kind of sleepy boredom that makes you hunch over in a dark theater or on a long bus ride, and gravity. Gravity?

Ah, gravity. That pesky downward tug of the

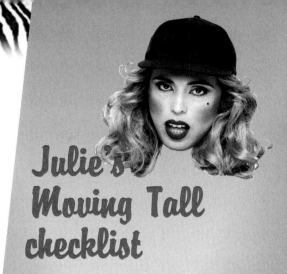

Julie's Moving Tall checklist

Head: Keep chin up and look straight ahead.

Neck: Hold it elongated, relaxed, and centered between your shoulders.

Shoulders: Relax them backward and down by opening your chest and keeping your rib cage lifted.

Arms: Bend naturally, at a 90-degree angle. Move your arms close to your body so your hands are level with your chest at the top of the swing and down to your hipbones at the bottom.

Hands: Cup gently. Pretend you're holding a butterfly in each palm and you don't want to crush the poor little things.

Abs: Lift up tall. Pull them in toward your spine.

Lower Back: Maintain a natural arch, or a slight inward curve. This varies from person to person, but no person should let their butt stick out. This means your back is too arched.

Hips: Stay loose and relaxed. Hips should move forward, not side to side.

Legs: Extend them fully but don't lock your knees. Remember, your stride is powered from your hip and torso, not just from your legs.

Feet: Land firmly, heel first, toe flexed up toward your shin. Roll through your heel to your arch, to the ball of your foot, to your toes. Push off your toes rather than pounding off the entire length of your foot.

SLEEP STRAIGHT

Now that you've got this plethora of peppy posture information in your head that you keep trying to remember, thank goodness you can go to sleep and forget all about it. Don't pull the covers over your eyes just yet, sweetie. Believe it or not, your sleeping posture has a huge impact on your standing, sitting, moving, and other wide-awake postures. Have you ever noticed how stiff you feel when you first wake up in the morning? Whether you tossed and turned or slept like a rock, conditions like backaches and neck-aches often feel worse first thing in the morning. This may be related to both the way you sleep and what you're sleeping on. So before you get a visit from Mr. Sandman tonight, here are a few things you should consider:

Sleep in the position that's most comfortable for you. However, the most posture-enhancing position, and the one that's healthiest for your lower back, is on your side with your knees bent and your head supported on a low pillow. Piling up pillows may cause neck strain because your neck muscles must work all through the night to keep your head propped up.

When sleeping on your back, put a pillow under your knees. This is for support; again, use a low pillow.

Have a firm mattress if you sleep on your stomach. Sleeping on your stomach has long been thought to increase your lower-back curve and, thus, lower-back pain. If you must do it, make sure your mattress is very firm and your pillow very low so your head remains close to the level of your shoulders. Make sure that your mattress has no dead or sagging spots and that the coils are springy. If not, replace it.

Don't let the bedbugs bite. Follow these very simple guidelines, have sweet dreams, and wake up less stiff and more cheerful.

earth that binds the stars and planets together and keeps you planted on the ground. When you're young, you're busy developing those rotten postural habits, but at least you don't have much trouble carrying your share of the gravitational load. As you get older, it gets harder and harder to literally carry the weight of the world on your shoulders. Like a slow-acting trash compactor, gravity gradually compresses your spine, drags your shoulders forward, and distorts your postural curves; by the time you reach seventy, you can expect to shrink a few inches in height.

Bad Strategies, Good Strategies

Typically, your body responds to all of this environmental stimuli and trauma by devising dysfunctional strategies. One problem is kyphosis, or rounded, droopy shoulder, which causes chronic neck pain. Another is lordosis, a case of excessively arching your lower back like a sway-backed horse. This results in lower-back discomfort. Another is scoliosis, or a sideways curvature of the spine, which leads to all types of physical difficulties.

Your body can take one of these coping strategies to the extreme; a hunchback is just a really bad case of kyphosis. Most of us exhibit more minor incarnations, like a lower back that's a teensy bit overarched or a slightly sideways carriage. However, sooner or later off posture—even if it's only a little off—can lead to all sorts of nasty aches and pains. Did you know that more than 80 percent of adult Americans experience some sort of neck or back discomfort? You probably did, because you're probably one of them. Problems can range from a little twinge in the neck every now and then to really severe back pain that keeps you in bed for weeks at a time. According to medical and fitness experts, most of it is due to tight, weak muscles and a spine that's light-years away from ideal alignment.

What to do? Bring things back into balance. Put those freethinking vertebrae in their place. Teach those slackers who's boss. Straighten up. Realign yourself. Strengthen and lengthen your abdominal and back muscles which are responsible for both moving and supporting your spine. Learn to move with good alignment. Sounds easy, right? But how do you do it? The seven exercises described at the end of this chapter can help realign and rebalance your postural patterns; however, they're only part of the solution. You must also reprogram the way you stand, sit, move. When you stand, review the points in the "Stand Up for Good Posture" section, right. When you sit, especially at your desk, make sure you follow the advice we give you in "Ergonomic Correctness" on pages 132–133. When you walk, run, or otherwise locomote, review the "Moving Tall Checklist" on page 129 every fifteen minutes or so. Hell, we even give you advice on good sleeping posture on page 130. After a while, you'll find you won't have to think about your posture points so often, because they'll become your new and improved postural habits.

This may seem like a lot to remember, but it's a great way to unpack all that baggage you've got. In other words, an entire lifetime of ingrained poor posture habits. Feeling guilty about how bad slouching is? Don't be so hard on yourself; there are spine-strengthening exercises starting on page 135.

Stand Up for Good Posture

When you stand with good posture, you appear relaxed and balanced. Here's what it should look like:

- Your head is centered between your shoulders and your shoulders are square.

- Your chest is broad and open, your rib cage lifted.

- Your abs are gently pulled inward toward your spine and your tailbone points toward the floor.

- Your knees are soft and "unlocked" and your weight is evenly distributed on both of your feet.

That's not too much to ask, is it? Well, it must be, because most of us don't stand up straight.

Ergonomic Correctness

Like nail biting or gum snapping, lousy posture is simply an ingrained behavioral pattern. You can teach yourself to change. A major step to revamping posture involves proper ergonomics, which is just a fancy word for setting up your work environment for maximum efficiency and comfort.

So many of us hold jobs that are sedentary and also highly repetitive. We sit all day repeating over and over again a particular pattern of movement that generally occurs in a small amount of space and uses only a few, select muscle groups. Let's take typing. When you type, your fingers and wrists travel a centimeter or so up and down, up and down, for hours on end. Eventually, they feel achy and sore even when you're not banging away at a keyboard; your back and shoulders also feel achy and sore from slouching forward too long.

The trouble is, *Homo sapiens* were never meant to sit around for long stretches of time. They were designed to hunt, gather, chop, dig, and climb. Well, this is the information age, pal. Hunting, gathering, chopping, digging, and climbing can get you arrested. In any case, these activities don't really get you ahead in the job market anymore unless you're in tabloid journalism, where this behavior is encouraged, nurtured, and rewarded.

Realistically, you're probably going to have to adjust to your office environment because you're probably stuck with it for a few more years. We have some suggestions on how to make it a more ergonomically friendly place to hang out.

- Choose a chair that supports your back. If your chair doesn't have decent back support, get another one or, at the very least, purchase a lumbar roll that fits between the small of your back and the back of your chair. As a temporary measure, you can use a rolled-up bath towel.

- Adjust your chair so your knees are level with your hips and your feet are flat on the floor. If that isn't possible with your current chair, place a book or two underneath your feet.

- Center yourself in front of your computer screen so you're about two feet away and looking directly at it or slightly up. This prevents slouching and leaning.

- Place your keyboard so your arms hang loosely at your sides and your elbows remain at right angles. Keep your wrists in line with your forearm and maintain a

which shoes fit your spine?

Shoes that don't offer the proper cushioning can result in back pain. Shoes that don't offer the proper ventilation can result in a really bad stink.

light touch on the keyboard. You may want to experiment with one of those new ergonomically correct keyboards with the revamped key configurations. It may take you a while to become familiar with key placement and moving your fingers to different places but they really do eliminate problems.

■ Don't cradle the receiver between your ear and shoulder when you're talking on the phone. If you spend a lot of time on the phone, you should probably consider a headset. Although you might feel like "Amy the Time-Life Operator" or like you're on your "Blonde Ambition" tour or like you should ask someone if they'd like a hot apple or cherry pie with their meal, you'll eliminate much of the wear and tear on your neck.

■ Most important, sit up straight. You don't look as much like you have a broomstick up your ass as you think you do! Seriously, don't round your lower back! It helps to get up from time to time when you work, just to remind yourself that you can. It will do wonders for both your back and your spirit.

Spinal Rx

It's often the case with back pain that you feel worse if you take to your bed; this weakens the very muscles that need to be loosened and strengthened and does nothing to help the vertebrae fall back into their correct placement. Another traditional treatment, the heating pad, makes many back conditions worse by further inflaming the nerves. So what spells relief for an aching back?

Time, for one thing. Many cases of back pain disappear within four weeks without any treatment at all. If that doesn't work, you can see a variety of professionals. Most experts believe that the majority of back pain is muscular in nature and can be treated successfully with nonsurgical procedures like stretching, strengthening, massage, physical therapy, and chiropractic. (To avoid the chiropractic quacks, make sure you get a good recommendation from a friend or, better yet, from a medical doctor.) Some doctors treat back pain as if it is psychosomatic; they'll tell you the pain is all in your head—well, in your back—and if you'd just learn how to relax it would all go away. Swimming, walking, and yoga seem to be the best activities for limbering up tight back muscles. Exercises like the ones in this chapter and in the "Guts!" chapter are also helpful.

For a lower-back episode you're having *right now,* ice and gentle movement will probably give you the most relief. Some experts recommend seeing a physiatrist, a medical doctor who specializes in disabilities. If you experience severe back pain that prevents you from going about your normal activities, see your general practitioner to rule out any underlying medical causes, like kidney infections or intestinal disorders, that often list back pain as a symptom.

If you have neck pain of the non-whiplash-due-to-a-car-accident kind, this usually signals tightness in the muscles of your neck, upper back, and/or shoulders. One remedy is to gently stretch your neck muscles. Massage is also very useful for freeing up knotty neck muscles. Ice, usually an injury-friendly treatment, isn't always the best choice for neck pain. If you're stiff to begin with, applying ice may cause you to tense up even more. Moist heat in the form of a warm washcloth, shower massage, or whirlpool is the way to go for a simple case of stiff neck.

Seven Exercises to Reboot Your Posture

Here are seven posture exercises you can do every day if you want to. To see real differences in the way you hold yourself, you'll need to do them regularly at least twice a week. On the days when you're doing your regular workout anyway, do them at the end of your workout. If all you're doing are these exercises, warm up with 3–5 minutes of easy aerobic activity like the old marching in place or the old pedaling on an exercise bike (as mentioned in the chapter "Move!" and rementioned in the chapter "Pump!").

If you do 5–15 repetitions of each exercise, the entire routine should take about 10 minutes. Count on spending a little more time when you're first learning them. Do the exercises in the order they're listed; that way, each move flows right into the next and you don't have to keep rolling over, sitting up, and lying back down again.

Obviously, if something bothers your lower back or neck or anywhere else, don't ignore the pain. Stop immediately. Reread the exercise description and look at the accompanying photo to make sure you're doing everything right. If you feel you're doing the move correctly and it still causes discomfort—skip it. Try it again after you've been working out consistently for a few months; pain in the spine is often just a lack of strength and/or flexibility.

back pain

Ever notice how you never notice how often you use your back until it hurts? That's when you find out you use it for every single thing you do: sleeping, walking, sitting, running, driving, making love, making excuses. We have ways to give you back your back.

Rolling Like a Ball

Have a ball stretching, massaging, and rebalancing your spine!

The Setup Sit up tall and hug your knees into your chest by loosely clasping a hand around each ankle. Drop your head between your knees and pull your abs in toward your spine. Point your toes and lift your feet an inch or so off the floor so that you are balanced evenly on the center of both buttocks.

The Move Pull your abs even further into your spine and shift your weight backward so you roll backward as far as your shoulder blades. Shift your weight forward and roll up once again into the balanced position. Hold a moment before rolling back again.

Thinking with Your Muscles Control the movement with your abdominals, *not* with momentum. You're doing this move correctly if you roll easily up into the balanced position and are able to hold it without a lot of wiggling around.

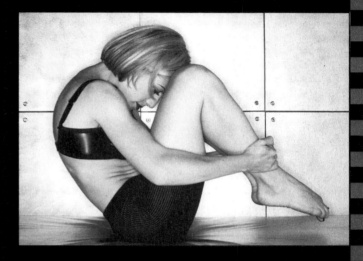

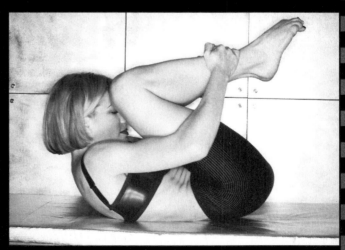

Pelvic Tilts

Stretches and strengthens the lower back, buttocks, abs, and hamstrings! A great spine realigner!

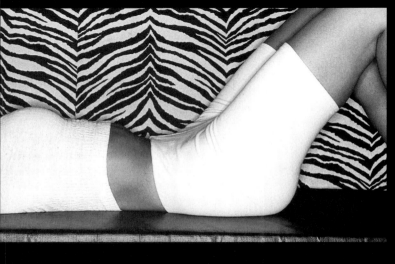

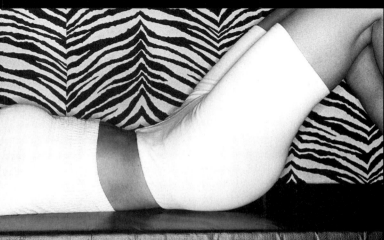

The Setup Lie on your back with your knees bent, feet flat on the floor and hip width apart. Lace your hands together and place them underneath your head. Anchor your back to the floor by pulling your abdominals in toward your spine.

The Move Gently squeeze your buttocks together and tilt your hipbones up until your buttocks curl 1–2 inches upward off the floor. Hold a moment and slowly lower to the start.

Thinking with Your Muscles Your lower back should remain anchored to the floor throughout the movement. You'll feel a contraction in your buttocks, abs, and hamstrings and a stretch in your lower back as you tilt upward. Make sure you don't arch your back off the floor when you lower to the start.

The Swimmer

Realigns the spine and strengthens the upper and middle back, shoulders, and abdominals!

The Setup Lie face down with your arms stretched out in front of you, palms down, fingers pointing forward, and your legs straight out behind you, buttocks squeezed gently together, toes softly pointed. Pull your abdominals inward and tilt your pelvis downward until there is a small space between your stomach and the floor. Keeping your arms straight, lift them a few inches off the floor and gently squeeze your shoulder blades together.

The Move Make a slow, wide circle with your arms until they are behind your back. Clasp one hand in the other. Lift your chest off the floor as you stretch your arms toward your feet. Slowly circle back and lower your body to the start.

Thinking with Your Muscles Imagine you're stroking through the water. Concentrate on extending and stretching the entire length of your body. You'll feel this exercise in the upper back and shoulders.

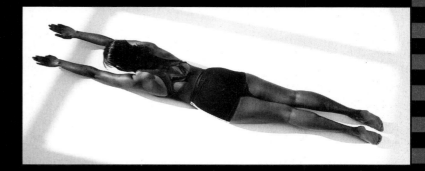

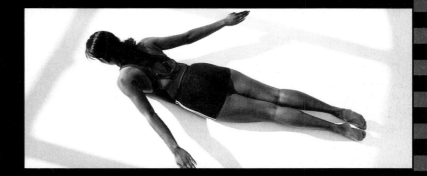

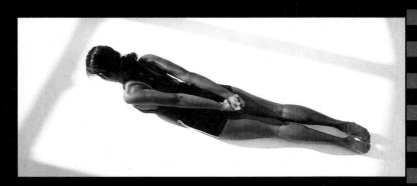

Cat Cow

A groovy way to stretch the lower back and abs and loosen up the spine!

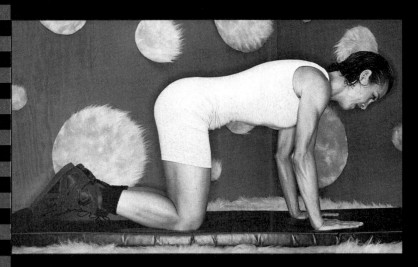

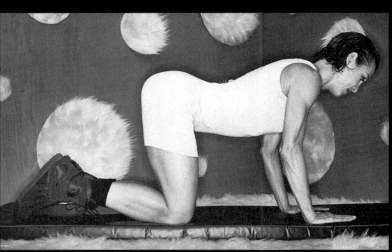

The Setup Start on all fours on a padded surface with your knees hip width apart and your arms shoulder width apart, weight balanced evenly on your hands and feet. Look down at the floor so that the back of your neck is lengthened and in line with the rest of your spine.

The Move Moving slowly, pull your abs in toward your spine and arch your back upward; hold a moment and then gently drop your back and abdominals downward.

Thinking with Your Muscles As you round up (cat), you'll feel a stretch from your neck all the way through your lower back; as you drop downward (cow), you'll feel your abdominals lengthen and your lower back loosen up. Don't exaggerate either movement.

Horse Biting Tail

Super for stretching your spine laterally, thus increasing freedom of movement!

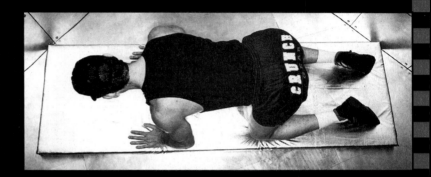

The Setup Start on all fours on a padded surface with your knees hip width apart and your arms shoulder width apart, weight balanced evenly on your hands and feet. Look down at the floor so that the back of your neck is lengthened and in line with the rest of your spine; pull your abs inward.

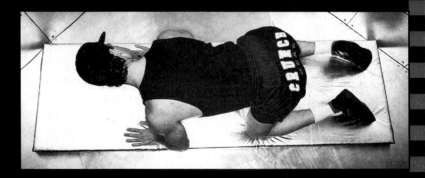

The Move Look over your right shoulder and twist your right hip toward your head until you can just see your right foot (or as far as you can comfortably twist). Hold for about 10 seconds and then slowly return to the center before twisting to the left. Alternate sides.

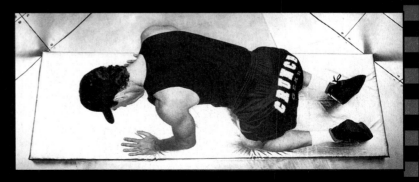

Thinking with Your Muscles You'll feel a good stretch travel along the curve of your spine, especially if you concentrate on keeping your abdominals pulled inward and your weight balanced evenly on all fours.

Finding Your Links

Great for stretching the backs of thighs! Makes your whole spine feel better!

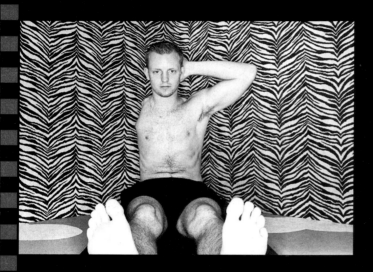

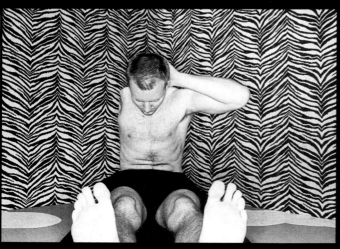

The Setup Sit up tall with your legs out in front of you and comfortably apart. Gently flex your feet. Place your hands behind your head, palms against your scalp, fingertips touching, and extend your elbows out wide. Pull your abs in toward your spine and drop your chin to your chest.

The Move Pull your abs inward even more and round your back as much as you comfortably can. Hold a moment and then slowly, one vertebra at a time, straighten up to the start so you are sitting up very tall. Hold a moment before rerounding your back and beginning the next rep.

Thinking with Your Muscles The goal of this exercise is to "find the link" from one vertebra to the next. Roll up as slowly as possible; try to feel each vertebra stack directly on top of the one beneath it. Don't force either the rounding or the straightening phase of the stretch and concentrate on keeping your elbows wide throughout the movement.

The Wall Roll-up

A cool way to readjust alignment while you make your back and abs more powerful!

The Setup Stand with your entire back against a wall, feet flat and about 6 inches out in front of you, hip width apart. Let your arms relax down at your sides. Press the entire length of your back firmly into the wall by squeezing your shoulder blades together, tilting your hipbones slightly forward, and pulling your abs in toward your spine.

The Move Starting at the neck, slowly moving one vertebra at a time, peel your back off the wall and lean forward. When your entire back, up to your tailbone, has come off the wall, hang for a moment, allowing your arms and shoulders to relax and go limp, and then curl back up to the start pressing one vertebra at a time back into place.

Thinking with Your Muscles Think of your vertebrae as a zipper you're trying to slowly open as you roll down and close as you roll up. If you feel any pain in your lower back, only roll as far forward as is comfortable.

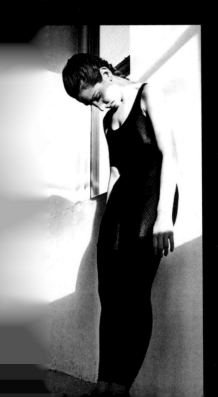
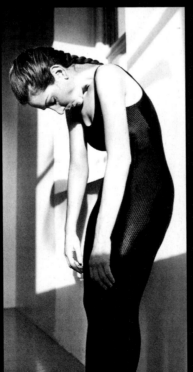
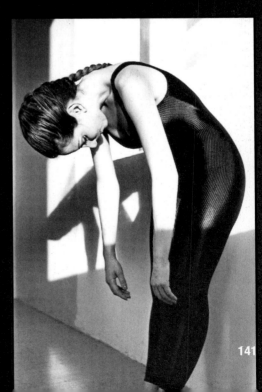

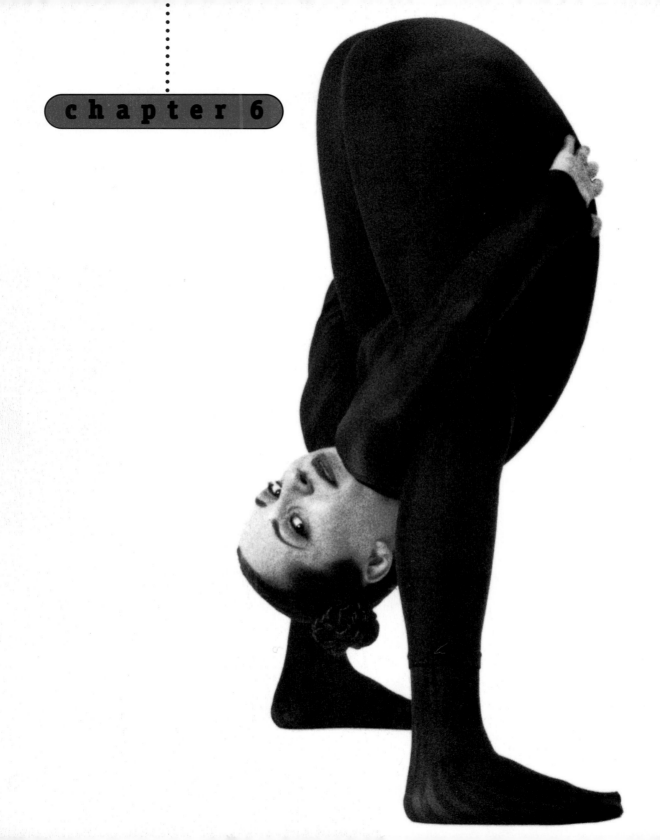

stretch!

Stretching for Flexibility and Injury Prevention

Can you suck your toes? If so, you may have a career in film ahead of you. If not, ever wonder why babies can do it and you can't? Well, their muscles and bones aren't fully developed; nor are they taxed by activities that make them tight and stiff. So how do we go from being precocious little mini-contortionists to creaky, inflexible grown-ups? First you have to understand what flexibility really is.

Flexibility is the range of motion or distance a joint can move. It's the maximum you can reach, twist, swing, flex, extend, or bend a part of your body. By the time you hit your early twenties, your bones have hardened, your joints have set in place. So while you lose the ability to suck your toes like little Popsicles, you do gain a certain

amount of stability because bones and muscles stay put inside their joint sockets (barring any traumatic incidents to your joints, of course).

However, along with this stability often comes a certain degree of inflexibility. Due to misuse, disuse, and injury, your joints stiffen, your muscles shorten and tighten. When you bend over in an attempt to tie your shoelaces and only make it as far as your knees,

double-jointed lies

People who can do splits are not double-jointed; they just have flexible ligaments. There's no such thing as having two joints in the same location. Hope you haven't told lots of people you're double-jointed.

These Crunch members put their hands in the air like the bank robber off-camera tells them to. Okay, seriously—they enjoy stretching exercises with their Crunch instructor.

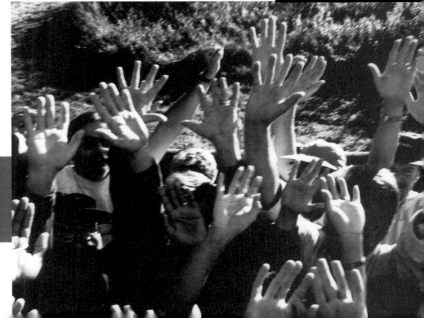

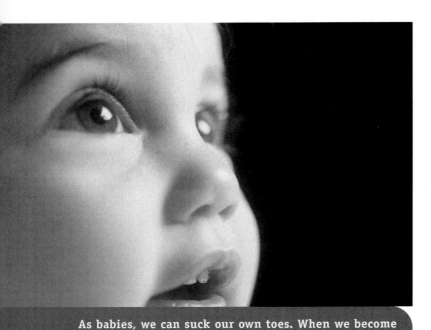

As babies, we can suck our own toes. When we become creaky adults, other people must suck our toes for us.

it's the lack of flexibility in your lower back and the backs of your thighs, as well as in the muscles attached to these joints, which prevents you from making it all the way down to shoelace level.

The longer you neglect the situation, the worse things get. Before you know it, you wake up one day feeling like the Tin Man before Dorothy and Toto came along: stiff, tight, rusted, and whiny. But you don't need an oilcan. You need stretching.

Stretching involves getting into a position and holding it long enough to give your muscles a chance to relax and elongate. Because muscles have an elastic

quality—they stretch out but spring back into shape much like a rubber band—you must hold each stretch long enough for it to retain some of its stretched length and you must do this often enough so your muscles remember to stay permanently elongated. Don't worry. You'll learn more about that later.

In a way, stretching a muscle does the exact opposite of strengthening it. The goal of strength training is to make the muscle contract, or shorten, in order to overcome a resistance; the goal of stretching is to make the muscle relax and lengthen to overcome a tension. Strength gives your muscles the ability to handle more work; stretching makes your muscles more supple and pliable.

And, contrary to popular belief, your strength training will not limit your flexibility or make you "muscle-bound." In fact, if you train properly and work every exercise through using a complete and natural range of motion, your flexibility should actually improve. Natural range of motion in an exercise like the Shoulder Press on page 71 means lowering the weights to your shoulders and then straightening your arms up till your elbows are slightly bent but not completely locked. The more you work out, the more you'll get a feel for the natural range of each exercise and also your body's flexibility abilities.

Stretching Is Not a Scientific Matter

Though most experts, top athletes, and professional dancers are convinced regular stretching prevents injury and eases the muscular soreness caused by overdosing on other forms of exercise, this has never been proven. Enhanced flexibility doesn't seem to improve athletic performance either, at least in studies that looked at world-class runners. However, one thing is clear: You need a certain amount of mobility to comfortably perform the everyday stuff. Remember those shoelaces you couldn't tie? Or the trouble you have straightening up to full height? Or that itch on your shoulder blade you can't quite reach? Stretching helps

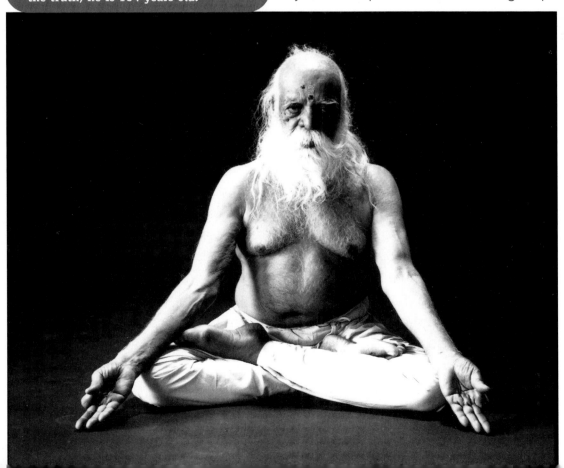

Swami stretches in the yoga classes he teaches. And unless Swami is stretching the truth, he is 104 years old.

145

you achieve and maintain the amount of flexibility you need to perform these mundane but necessary chores.

Besides, stretching feels good when you do it correctly. It's the perfect antidote to all that pumping and pounding we do. And what better way to transition out of stress mode than a few minutes of gentle, easy stretching? Stretching-type disciplines such as yoga and tai chi have been used as forms of meditation for thousands of years.

Yo, I Ain't No Nadia Comaneci

Everyone has a different capacity for flexibility. Gymnasts, with their full splits onto thin wooden beams, are on one end of the spectrum, while those of us who have trouble getting out of bed in the morning are on the other. Flexibility may also vary from one joint to the next. Your shoulders may be loose enough to allow you to clasp your hands behind your back but your neck may still be tight. That's why it's so important to thoroughly stretch all your major muscle groups, including your legs, lower back, chest, upper back, shoulders, and arms.

As with any other physical parameter, genetics, fitness level, and skill will dictate how much you can influence the mobility and pliability of your joints and muscles. For some people, it comes easy. For others, it's like someone poured cement into your joint sockets; you'll have to work a little harder at it, but don't get discouraged. Everyone can improve their flexibility. In fact, most people notice a difference after their very first stretching session. You don't need to dedicate your entire life to stretching if your aim is simply to loosen up a bit and move around a little more freely. Five to ten minutes a day should be more than enough to get the job done.

Your Body Will Let You Know Your Limits

How much should I stretch? You really have to listen to your body rhythms. You'll have days when you feel tighter than a size 3 spandex dress and your body makes a lot of snaps, crackles, and pops. Then you'll have other days when you're really loose. If you pay attention to your body's day-to-day flexibility level, you'll know when to push it and when to hang back a bit. You'll probably find that you'll make remarkable progress for a few weeks and then none at all for the next month. That's okay. Stretching is not something you should stress about when the whole point is to make you feel good. So don't force the issue if your body rhythms aren't right.

12 Steps to Stretching

Before you begin the stretching routine in this chapter, take some time to review the basic principles of flexibility training.

1 Stretch after your workout, not before.
It doesn't matter what you've heard or what you've done in the past, here's the final word on when to stretch: after your workout, not before. Stretching is not a warm-up. It is more in the cooldown area. Warming up is getting your blood flowing and raising your body temperature with a rhythmic, aerobic type of activity like walking, jogging, cycling, light stepping, or calisthenics. Warm-up activities, besides reducing the risk of injury and delaying muscle soreness, also makes your muscles more receptive to stretching.

2 Hold each position between 10 and 60 seconds.
This gives the muscle time to stretch beyond its normal resting length and retain some of its newly acquired elasticity. If you're a stretching neophyte, begin with the minimum holding time and gradually work your way up to the full 60 seconds.

3 Don't bounce or make jerky movements.
Doing this may actually make you tighter. All stretching should be done slowly and smoothly with the minimum of unnecessary fussing and futzing. Get into the proper stretching position and stay there. Then, after you've held the stretch for a few seconds, slowly move further into it.

4 Never force a stretch.
A stretch should feel like a mild-to-strong pull that gradually travels the length of the muscle as you hold a position. Stretch to a point where you're right on the edge of discomfort but never to the point of "ouch!"

5 Breathe deeply and naturally.
This increases your flexibility by helping you to mellow out and by sending oxygen-rich blood speeding into your muscles. Inhale deeply just before you go into a stretching position and then exhale through your mouth as you

afternoon delight

Muscles become easier to stretch after they've warmed up. Thus, flexibility peaks at about 6 P.M., making the late afternoon and evening the best time for stretching. Workaholics: Stop cringing. Take a stretching break and go back to work.

move into it. Breathe deeply several times as you hold the stretch.

6 Tighten the muscle opposite to the one you're stretching.

Find the muscle located opposite to the one you're stretching and contract or tighten it. Tightening the opposing muscle group creates an equal and opposite reaction in the muscle being stretched, so the more you tighten on one side of the joint, the better you are able to stretch the other side. For instance, if you're stretching your hamstring (located in the back of your thigh), then at the same time tighten your quadriceps (the muscle in the front of your thigh). Many people call this reciprocal inhibition or active isolated stretching. Both are fancy terms for enhancing your muscle's ability to relax and lengthen.

7 Think with your muscles.

Yes, the old "think with your muscles"— a recurring theme in the book, we know. Luckily computers have "copy" and "paste" for repeated phrases such as this, right? The fact is, however, that you can't just go through the motions and say, "There! I've stretched!" You must always focus on what you're do-

ing and think with your muscles. For example, do you feel the stretch where you're supposed to? Is your form correct? Should you back off or push a little further? It's not enough to make the shape of the exercise. You've got to tune in to the muscle you're stretching.

8 Listen for muscular mutterings.

If your muscle is being pushed too hard, or isn't responding, tune in and listen. If it tells you to modify your move to make it easier, then do it. It's telling you to back off and it means it. Remember, it can always get you back— pulled muscles, torn muscles, strained muscles are realities. So listen up. You can always go back to a harder stretch after a few weeks of regular flexibility training and try it again.

9 Stretch muscles from different angles.

When you do the Hamstring Stretch (the third stretch in our routine), you may want to turn your toe out slightly to emphasize the inside of the back of your thigh. It's cool to experiment by slightly changing the angle of any of the stretches you try so long as you remember the "no pain" rule.

148

10 **Stretch the muscles you use most.**

Give priority to the muscles you use the most in your workout and in everyday life, but don't neglect any major muscle group. Example: Cyclists should pay extra attention to the flexibility of their thighs, calves, and lower back but shouldn't skip upper-body stretches altogether. Your goal should be total, full-body flexibility. Our stretching routine is designed to stretch all of your main muscles.

11 **To remain flexible, you have to keep stretching.**

Your muscles will "remember" to stay loose and flexible if they're reminded often enough . . . so be consistent. We recommend stretching after every workout, or, if you can, every single day.

12 **Don't make a contest out of stretching.**

This is not about seeing who can touch their tongue to their shoulder blade. There's no optimum amount of flexibility, only what's ideal for you. Contortionists are people who have been stretching to an extreme, generally since they were children. As for you, just stretch within the limits and abilities of your individual joints and muscles.

Routine Stretching

Here's a series of stretches for you to try. This routine was designed to stretch all the major areas of your body. Do them in order and you'll find that each move flows directly into the next. We've designed the routine so you only do one of each stretch, but if you feel particularly fond of one, go ahead and do it two or three times. What a great way to relax!

Be sure to read the 12-step approach to stretching. You'll find out how long to hold each stretch, what proper stretching feels like, and much, much more. If you haven't read it already, don't forget to do it before you start stretching.

The stretches we've given you are not the only stretches in the world, just as the strengthening and aerobic exercises we describe in other chapters aren't the only ones in the world. But we think they're good ones. Try 'em out and do the whole routine or just the ones you like. Go through some stretching books or go to a stretch class and add some more. Pretty soon, you'll be a stretching junkie.

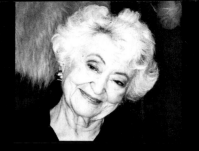

This is Rosie Feldman, grandmother of the photographer. She's 95 and still exercising like nobody's business. When Rosie can't get a Swedish massage, she opts for the Double Knee Hug.

Double Knee Hug

A gentle massage for your lower back!

The Setup Lie flat on your back. Hug your knees in close to your chest. Make sure to allow your head and shoulders to remain easy, relaxed, and loose.

The Move As you hug your knees in toward your chest, gently tighten your embrace. Continue this exercise for one more minute. A minute might seem like a long time but doing it this long should make you feel good.

Thinking with Your Muscles This relaxing move should feel like a gentle massage on your lower back. You can do this stretch as part of your ab routine or anytime your back feels tight or sore.

Easier Only hug one knee into your chest at a time.

Harder Gently rock your hips from side to side and roll them in small circles.

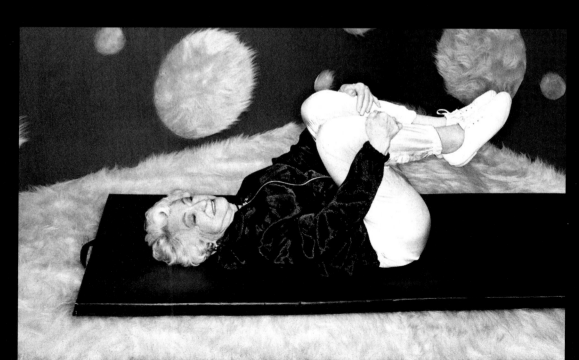

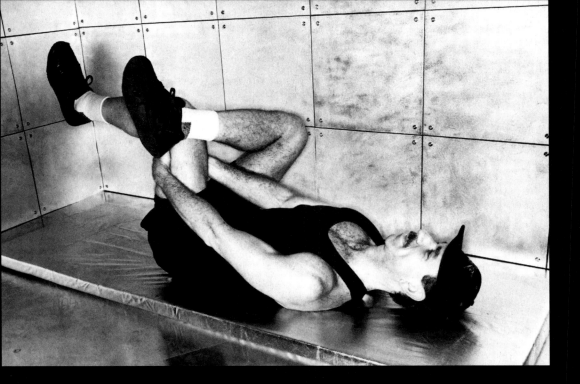

The Pretzel

Stretches your buttocks and lower back!

The Setup Lie on your back with your left knee bent, foot flat on the floor. Cross your right ankle over your left thigh. Keep your back flat on the floor and your entire spine (including your neck) aligned.

The Move Lift your foot off the floor and raise your leg until your left thigh is directly over your hip. Clasp your hands around your left thigh and pull backward. Hold. Slowly lower to the floor, switch leg positions, and repeat.

Thinking with Your Muscles You'll feel a stretch in your right buttock when you pull back on your left leg and vice versa. You may also feel a mild stretch through your lower back.

Easier Pick your legs up off the floor without pulling backward on your thigh or pull backward with your outside hand only.

Harder Straighten your right leg upward as you pull back.

Hamstring Stretch

Great for backs of thighs! Makes your back feel better!

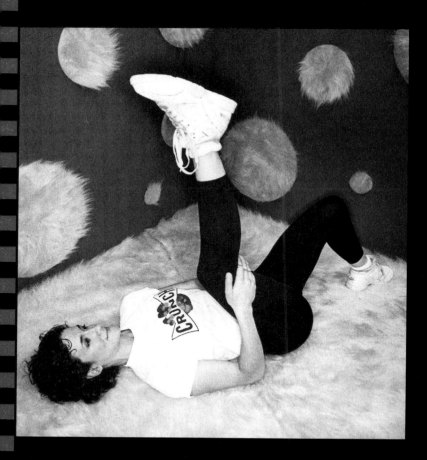

The Setup Lie on your back with your knees bent, feet flat on the floor, arms down at your sides, entire spine aligned.

The Move Keeping your knee slightly bent, raise your right leg up over your hip, or as far back as you can lift it without arching your lower back off the floor. Hold. Slowly lower to the start and repeat with your left leg.

Thinking with Your Muscles You'll feel a stretch gradually spread from the bottom of your butt to just behind your knee. If you feel pain or discomfort in your lower back, bend your knee a little more or discontinue the stretch.

Easier Clasp your hands around the back of your leg, just below your knee. Gently pull back on your leg.

Harder To stretch your calf at the same time, flex your foot so your toe angles downward.

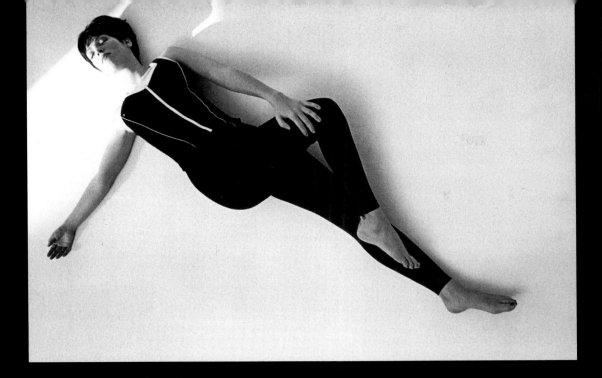

Hip Roll

Loosens up the entire spine plus your hips, butt, and outer thighs!

The Setup Lie on your back with your right knee bent, foot flat on the floor. Extend your left leg straight out along the floor. Place your hands wherever they're comfortable.

The Move Keeping your back and shoulders firmly anchored to the floor, roll your right hip off the floor and move your right knee across your body, pressing it to the left and downward. If possible, it should touch the floor on the left side. Pull your abs inward to return to the center; repeat to the other side.

Thinking with Your Muscles As you hold this position, the stretch will spread up into your shoulder and down into your lower back, hip, and buns.

Easier Bend both knees and drop them to one side, then the other.

Harder Place your left hand on the outside of your knee and gently apply downward pressure.

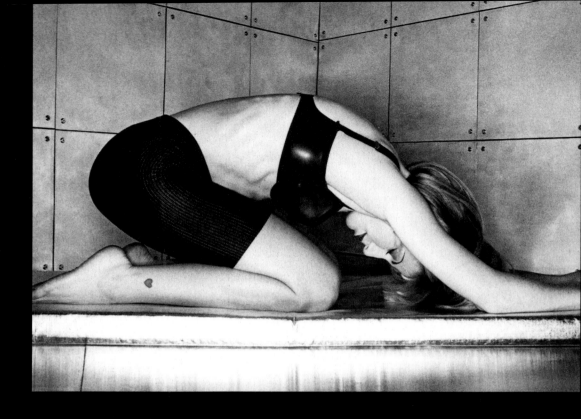

Back Release

Perfect for releasing tension all along your spine!

The Setup Kneel on your hands and knees with your entire spine aligned.

The Move Sit back onto your heels or as far back as you comfortably can. Hold.

Thinking with Your Muscles You'll feel a mild stretch along the length of your spine. This is an especially good stretch if your lower back is feeling a little tight or sore.

Easier Drop back only about halfway to your heels.

Harder Once you have stretched the middle of your spine, lean slightly to the right for a lateral stretch. Hold. Repeat to the left.

Cobra

Stretches your abdominals and the tops of your thighs!

The Setup Lie on your stomach with legs out straight, your arms bent, your weight resting on your elbows, and your hands clasped together. Place your forehead on the floor. Pull abs inward and tilt pelvis downward until hipbones make firm contact with the floor.

The Move Slowly lift your head and chest off the floor and press your weight even further into your elbows. Raise yourself as high as your flexibility allows without lifting hips off the floor. Lower to the start.

Thinking with Your Muscles You'll feel the stretch through the entire front of your torso all the way down to your thighs. If this hurts your lower back, don't press up as high or skip this one till you've worked on your back strength and flexibility for a while.

Easier Lift only your head off the floor.

Harder Straighten your arms up off the floor.

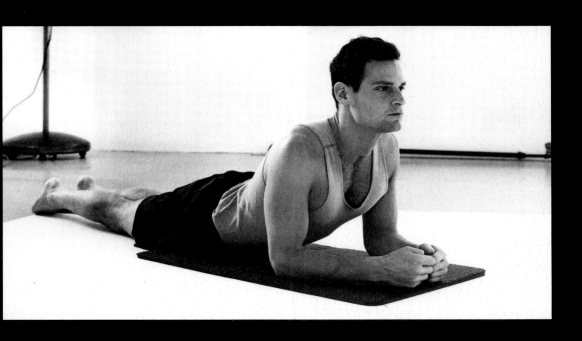

155

Half a Hug

Stretches your upper back, shoulders, and the fronts of your upper arms!

The Setup Sit up tall in a relaxed, comfortable position. Reach your right arm across your chest.

The Move Place the back of your left hand just in front of your elbow and gently press your arm toward your body. Hold. Repeat the stretch with your left arm.

Thinking with Your Muscles You'll feel the stretch in the back of your shoulder. It will gradually spread to your upper back and the entire length of your upper arm.

Easier Place the back of your left hand just behind your wrist.

Harder Place the back of your left hand behind your elbow.

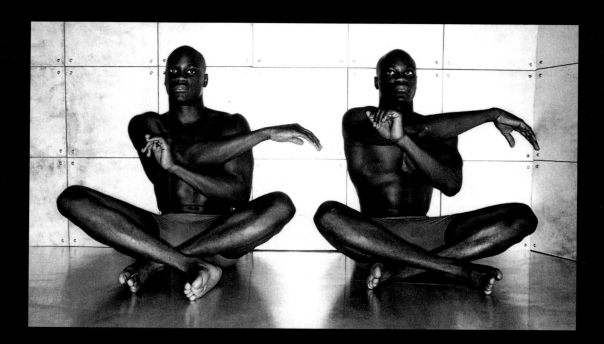

156

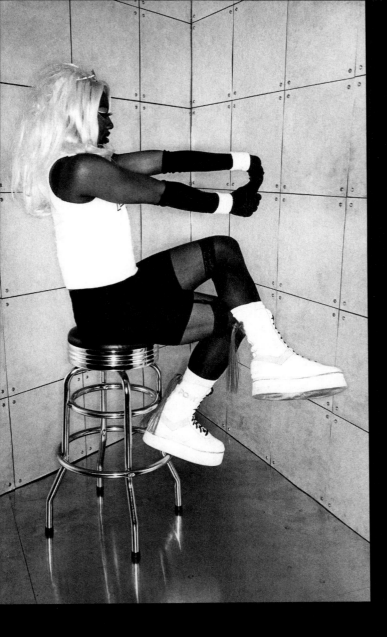

Forward Reach

Stretches your arm, wrist, and fingers!

The Setup Sit up tall in a relaxed, comfortable position. Extend your left arm in front of you up at shoulder height. Place the fingertips of your right hand over the fingertips of your left hand.

The Move Gently bend your left wrist downward and backward by applying a steady, even pressure on your fingertips. Hold. Repeat with your right arm.

Thinking with Your Muscles To start, you'll feel the stretch at the base of your wrist. As you hold, the stretch will spread up the length of your arm and down your fingertips.

Easier Make a loose fist with your left hand.

Harder Apply the pressure to the palm of your left hand.

157

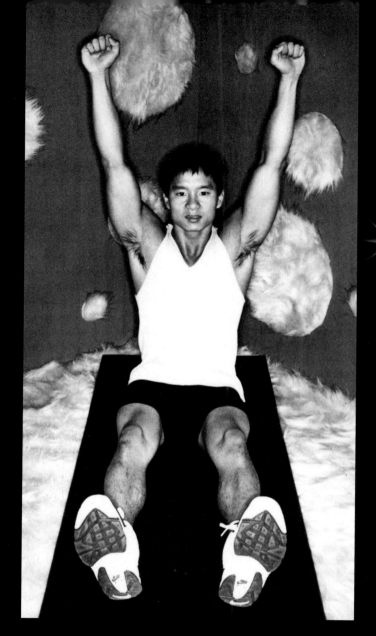

The Warrior

A super-duper stretch for your whole upper body and lower back!

The Setup Sit up tall with your legs straight out in front of you and comfortably apart. Make a loose fist with your hands and raise your arms directly over your shoulders.

The Move Lengthen your right arm upward as if trying to touch something above you that's just out of reach. Hold briefly. Without relaxing your right arm, reach your left arm upward. Sit up tall from the hips and keep your shoulders relaxed as you alternate stretching your arms upward five times on each side.

Thinking with Your Muscles The object is to pull up a little taller each time you stretch upward. You'll feel this stretch throughout the entire length of your spine, in the "wings" of your upper back, and in your shoulders and arms.

Easier Hold your arms a few inches forward rather than directly over your shoulders.

Harder After each stretch upward, press your arm a small distance backward.

Side Stretch

Stretches out your obliques, your spine, and your upper back!

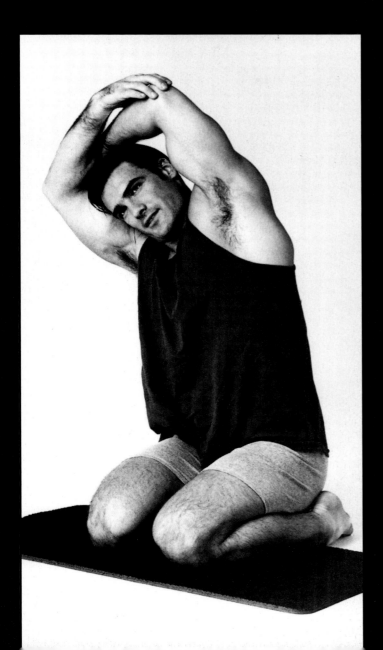

The Setup Sit up tall with your legs wherever they're most comfortable. Clasp one hand loosely in the other and raise your arms straight above your head.

The Move Lean to the right and reach your arms toward the opposite wall. Tip your head in the same direction. Hold briefly. Make sure you're sitting up tall from the hips and your shoulders are relaxed. Come back to the center and then stretch to the other side.

Thinking with Your Muscles You'll feel this stretch throughout the entire length of your spine, in the "wings" of your upper back, and in your shoulders and arms.

Easier If you find this too hard to do in any sitting position, try it standing.

Harder After each sideways stretch, press your arm a small distance backward.

Quad Stretch

Good for stretching your thighs and hips!

The Setup Lie on your left side with head resting on outstretched arm.

The Move Bend your right knee and lift your heel toward your buttocks. Grasp the top of your right foot with your right hand and gently press your heel even further into your buttocks. Hold. Repeat with your left leg.

Thinking with Your Muscles The stretch will originate at the top of your thigh just below your hip and gradually spread to the top of your knee.

Easier Lie on your side, bring your right heel to your buttocks, and grasp with your right hand.

Harder Hold higher up on the foot, near your ankle.

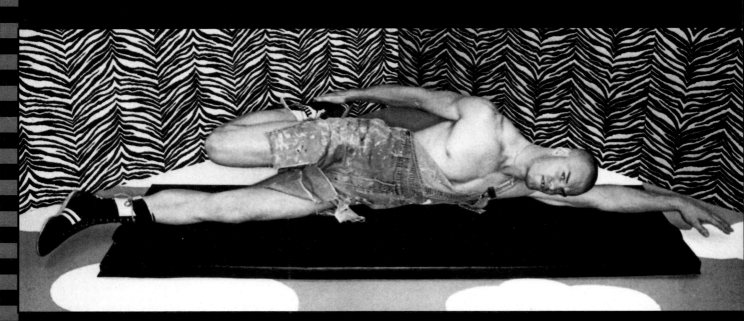

Wall Press

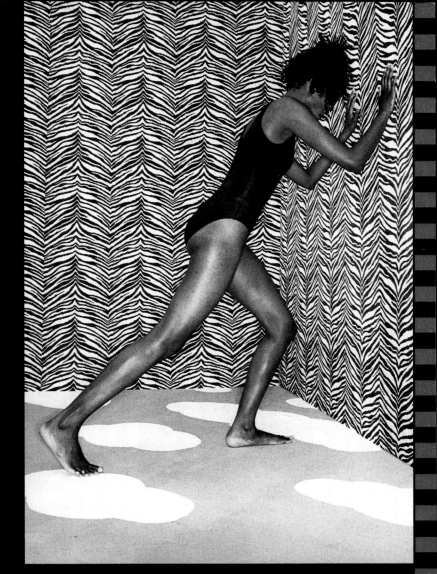

The Setup Stand an arm's length away from a wall and straddle your legs about 3 feet apart, left leg forward. Place the palms of your hands on the wall about shoulder width apart so your arms are straight with your elbows slightly bent.

The Move Bend your arms and left leg as you lean forward into the wall. Keeping your right leg straight, press your heel into the floor. Hold. Switch legs. Repeat.

Thinking with Your Muscles You'll feel the stretch spread through the length of your calf. It's okay if your heel doesn't make contact with the floor so long as you press it downward with steady, even pressure.

Easier Bend your right leg slightly as you press forward.

Harder Place your feet about hip width apart as you lean into the wall so you stretch both calves at the same time.

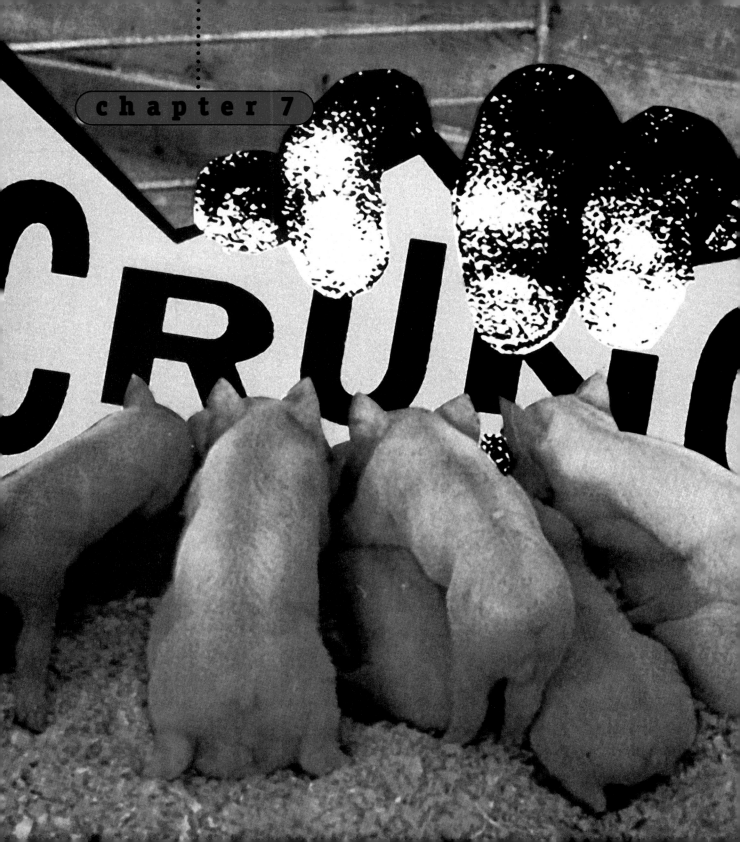

chow!

A Lesson in Nutrition, Fat, and Calorie Intake

Hard to Swallow

The acid from grapefruit helps "cleanse" your system and burn body fat. Eat ten eggs and a pound of bacon a day and the grease from these foods will cause excess fat to slide off your body. A serving of oat bran with every meal prevents calories from being absorbed. How many of these nutty too-good-to-be-true nutritional theories have you heard or read about and wanted so desperately to believe? They seem perfectly credible, since many such "new discoveries" are printed on the pages of some of the most respected periodicals in America.

It seems every nutritional study, no matter how flawed or bizarre, is announced to the public in a media frenzy. One day margarine is better for you than butter; the next day it's worse. Drinking caffeine suddenly is perfectly healthy; the next day kiss your wide-awake self good-bye. Drink a glass of red wine a day and you'll live longer; drink a glass of red wine a day and you'll die from liver problems . . .

It's like all these experts graduated with a Ph.D. in Indecision. Even if you make a sincere commitment to eating well, how can you know if you're eating well if those in the know don't even know?

The problem is, we're still learning about nutrition; new information comes to light every day. We'll try not to make things more confusing for you. Quality of life suffers when you're buried under information on how to live. No big serious diet menus. Just a little bit of generally accepted truisms about the stuff we eat and drink. Facts that were true for cavemen are true for you, and will be true for generations evolved enough to see all of mankind consistently put the seat down.

The subject of this chapter, "Chow!" or nutrition, is really just one of the five fitness factors we discussed in the chapter

"Flesh!" Because even if you follow all of our nutritional advice, and have the healthiest diet in the world, you won't be fit. Watching what you eat is just one thing you do in addition to aerobic exercise and strength training.

Nutrition 101

Energy from food is measured in calories. Your basal metabolic rate (BMR) is the number of calories you need per day just for basic bodily functions. BMR *only* takes into account the energy your body needs to run on autopilot; in other words, it covers the basics like the beating of your heart, the expansion and contraction of your lungs, the functioning of your liver, kidneys, and pancreas. It *does not* take into account any movement or exercise you happen to do during the day. For the average-sized woman, this number is around 1,000 calories; for the average-sized man, around 1,400. Movement generally raises average calorie need to around 1,600 and 2,000 for women and men, respectively. Exercise raises it even more.

You're more or less stuck with the BMR you're born with, but you can exert some influence over it. Exercise speeds up your metabolism, especially if you do enough of it to add muscle and drop body fat; some scientists speculate that a pound of muscle can increase your BMR by up to 50 calories a day.

Anyway, back to that 1,600-calorie-a-day diet for women. Maybe you think that number seems high, because diets tell you to restrict your intake to 800 to 1,000 calories a day in order to lose weight. The first time around, this strategy may work, but each time you reduce your calories below your BMR, your body, still programmed as it was millions of years ago, says, "Lazy man no bring home antelope again, save up calories for rainy day," and your metabolism lowers itself in response. So even though you're eating less, you may not lose weight. Studies seem to indicate that when you quit dieting (as most people inevitably do) your body bounces right back to its usual BMR, or set point; therefore, you're no better off weightwise than when you started. BMR, by the way, is also short for bummer.

This temporary metabolic work stoppage is a big reason why diets don't work. Of course, they also don't work because it's too uncomfortable to eat so little. As with a car with a nearly empty gas tank, there's too little fuel to run your organic engines properly. You feel hungry all the time and probably lack energy. (That's also why you often feel cold when you're dieting.)

Plus it's damn hard to stop eating the foods you love. Anytime you create an eating plan with an elaborate set of rules (good foods vs. bad foods and so on), you're doomed to failure. We're not saying you shouldn't aim for healthier eating habits, but you should be honest with yourself, and good to yourself too. If you absolutely, positively can't live without cherry cheesecake, better to have an occasional slice than binge on a whole cake every time your willpower caves in. Besides, as we learned in several other chapters, exercise can melt a lot of that cheesecake away. But the number of calories you take in and burn up is only part of the weight control and health picture. Where those calories come from is just as important.

Carbohydrates

People used to turn their noses up at simple foods even guys can cook, like spaghetti, potatoes, rice, and oatmeal. Now, they're considered the conquering heroes of nutrition. These starchy foods are good sources of carbohydrates, the nutrient most readily converted into glycogen. Remember from the "Move!" chapter that glycogen is the elementary fuel your body uses for life functions. It's used for everything from powering your muscle movements to maintaining your immune system.

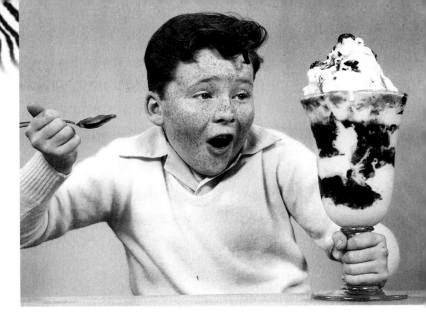

Though carbs should be the staple of any healthy diet, you have to be careful about the type of carbs you're talking about. There are complex carbs (starchy, bready, grainy foods, plus vegetables and legumes) and simple carbs (candy, cake, doughnuts, anything containing large amounts of sugar). Fruits, by the way, are a combination of complex and simple carbs; they're healthy because they contain lots of vitamins, minerals, fiber, and water.

Complex carbs are loaded with good stuff. Your body absorbs complex carbs slowly, so they provide a steady, even supply of energy. Simple carbs, on the other hand, are packed with empty, meaningless calories and are often found in foods that are also high in fat. They're absorbed quickly and affect your energy level like a roller coaster: a quick climb, followed by a quick drop. They're like a drunk uncle who

Once upon a time there was a diet that sounded too good to be true, which of course it always is.

The End.

(In nutrition, like everything else, the hardest thing to find is the truth.)

BMR: Basal Metabolic Rate is a very impressive way to describe the calories you burn not doing anything.

picks you up, throws you way up into the air, then drops you. When you eat a candy bar instead of lunch, you often feel groggy about a half hour afterward. This is an important rule about carbs, so listen up: Most of the calories you take in should come from complex carbs, about 60 percent. If you're very active, you may want to up your carb intake to 70 percent.

Protein

Muscles, organs, and blood are primarily composed of protein. Your body uses protein to build and repair these tissues and as a backup fuel supply when carbohydrates and fats aren't available. Proteins are made up of combinations of smaller building blocks called amino acids. There are twenty-two amino acids your body needs to function properly. Nine are called "essential" because you absolutely must get them from food; the other thirteen are termed "nonessential" because your body can produce them on its own. If you lack even one essential amino acid, your body will start breaking down muscle tissue to harvest the particular amino it needs. This is not an ideal situation. It can lead to things like hormonal imbalances and thin, fragile hair. Fortunately, this is a pretty rare occurrence these days. In fact, most of us get way *too much* protein.

So how much protein is enough but not too much? Only 15–20 percent of your calorie intake should come from protein sources like lean meats, poultry without skin, and fish. This translates into about 0.4 gram of protein per pound of body weight per day, or three modest servings of protein a day. (One serving of protein is about the size of a deck of cards.)

You can also get protein from many vegetables, soy, beans, and grains, but do keep in mind that most nonanimal protein sources are *incomplete;* that is, they contain some essential amino acids but lack others. Your body needs to have a specific assortment of amino acids present and accounted for at the same time in order to be able to make use of them. You can increase your chances of getting the right mix of aminos by combining your vegetarian protein sources. For instance, rice and beans will get you there. So will peanut butter on eight-grain bread and vegetarian chili and corn bread.

There's an old wives' tale that drinking protein shakes or eating a high-protein diet will help you bulk up your muscles because the extra protein is converted to muscle mass. In fact, researchers have found that the only people who may require additional protein are very lean endurance athletes who tend to metabolize their existing protein stores for energy during very long training sessions or in races. You don't need to up your protein intake if you're trying to build up or get stronger. A lot of bodybuilders think that's true, but it isn't. Even though your muscles are made of protein, your body's protein demands don't increase very much when you lift weights; any excess protein calories you take in will be either excreted or stored as unwanted body fat.

Fat

It's not just for fat people anymore. We all need a little fat. Fats are essential, providing vitamins and minerals you can't get from any other source. Fats insulate your body, padding and protecting your bones and organs. Fats furnish your body with the most efficient, abundant source of energy it has at its disposal. However, the average person eats a diet that's about 40 percent fat when they really should be eating more like 20–30 percent. Too much fat clogs your arteries and has been linked to heart disease and numerous types of cancer.

Now, 20 percent may be lower than you've previously heard quoted. Some organizations, including the American Heart Association, allow for a diet as high as 35 percent fat, but many experts don't think you can lose weight or maintain good health on a diet that high in fat. For one thing, it leaves no room for mistakes.

Even if you're careful to tally the amount of fat and calories in the foods you eat, you should know that the FDA still permits manufacturers a 20 percent margin of error in reporting the nutritional facts. So that 200-calorie muffin with 7 grams of fat may actually contain as many as 240 calories and 8 grams of fat. A 20 percent error over the course of days, weeks, and months can sabotage even the most diligent weight-loss efforts.

There are "good" fats and "bad" fats, although, strictly speaking, all fats are still fat. Just as there are "good" men and "bad" men, they're all still men. Saturated fats have all their chemical bonds fully stuffed with hydrogen ions (hence the name saturated). They're the true villains that muck up our diets by preventing the liver from filtering out LDL (low-density lipoprotein) cholesterol (otherwise known as "bad" cholesterol) from the blood. This raises both total cholesterol levels and levels of LDL cholesterol. Saturated fats are easy to recognize because they're all solid at room temperature; for example, the fat in your steaks or burgers, butter, cheese, avocado, and mayonnaise.

Most of your fats should be eaten in the form of monounsaturated and polyunsaturated fats. These "unsaturated fats" have the ability to liberate naturally occurring chemicals called free radicals into your bloodstream. In moderate amounts, free radicals have been shown to raise HDL (high-density lipoprotein) or "good," artery-cleansing cholesterol levels without increasing levels of LDL or "bad," artery-clogging cholesterol. Monounsaturates seem to be the most effective at cleaning up cholesterol levels because they lower the bad cholesterol without affecting the good cholesterol; these include olive oil and peanut oil. Polyunsaturates include sunflower, corn, and canola oils; although they do a good job of reducing bad cholesterol levels, they also lower levels of good cholesterol too. (More on cholesterol below.)

Since we brought it up at the beginning of the chapter, you probably want to know: "Is margarine a force of evil or just slippery, yellow, and misunderstood?" In moderate-to-small amounts, it's a good source of vitamins, but eating too much of it contributes to elevated cholesterol levels, especially if you're genetically disposed to high cholesterol. And consider this: Margarine is no different than butter in that it is pure fat. One small pat contains about 100 calories. A pat here, a pat there, and before you know it, your calorie intake is through the roof. There are some

recent indications (though who knows, that could change tomorrow) that margarine may have even more of a negative effect on your cholesterol level than butter. The moral? Use *all* fats sparingly.

Cholesterol

Animals produce cholesterol in their livers; hence animal fat is the only source of cholesterol. Since plants don't have livers, they don't produce cholesterol. Cholesterol, though a form of fat itself, doesn't contribute extra calories, but can affect your heart's health in a big, negative way by clogging your arteries, which can eventually lead to heart disease.

Here's a favorite trick manufacturers like to play regarding the fat and cholesterol contents of foods. It's possible for a food to be high in fat and low in cholesterol or vice versa. When a food label screams proudly, "Low in Cholesterol!!!!" look at the fine print carefully. There's a chance it's high in fat. Conversely, foods like lobster and shrimp are low in fat but outrageously high in cholesterol. Shrimp may have shrimpy livers but they still pump out the cholesterol.

As we already mentioned, there are two types of cholesterol: LDL and HDL. LDL is the substance that clings to the walls of your arteries, blocking them and forcing your heart to work harder to pump blood through your blood vessels. HDL cholesterol acts like a crew of maintenance workers; it scrubs your artery walls clean so blood has easy passage and your heart doesn't have to work as hard. You may have heard that you want your overall blood cholesterol to read 200 or lower but it's even more important to pay attention to your total cholesterol vs. HDL ratio; you want this ratio to be 5:1 or lower. For example, if your total cholesterol is 220 and your HDLs are 70, you divide 220 by 70, for a ratio of about 3:1. Although your total cholesterol number is a little high, it's balanced out by a high level of HDLs.

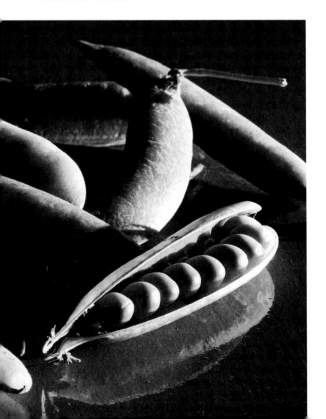

Fiber

Fiber is just a designer word for roughage, the indigestible residue of plant walls that helps cleanse your digestive system. In recent years, it's been shown to help lower cholesterol levels and prevent or at least reduce the risk of many types of cancer. Insoluble fiber absorbs water, thereby increasing bulk in your digestive system. This keeps things moving along through your intestines. Soluble fiber dissolves in water, so you fill up more quickly, possibly making weight control easier. It may help lower total cholesterol and blood pressure too. Grains, beans, fruits, and vegetables are good sources of insoluble fiber; whole oats and oat bran are the best sources of soluble fiber.

You need 20–35 grams of fiber daily to get its full effect. Most of us eat closer to 10 grams because we fill up on junk food and fast food which have had most or all of their natural fiber removed. Your best bet for increasing fiber intake is to eat foods closest to their natural state. Potatoes, for instance, are a pretty good source of fiber. But does it matter if we bake them, mash them, steam them, broil them, stick eyes, ears, and a nose on them, or fry them? Obviously, there's a big difference. A baked potato has 2.2 grams of fiber: By the time you peel it and mash it, you cut the fiber in half; once you cut it up and fry it, virtually all of the fiber disappears. Five half-cup servings a day of fresh fruits and vegetables plus three or four servings of whole-grain cereal or bread will easily meet your fiber requirements, but a word of caution: If you haven't had much experience with fiber, increase your intake gradually. Let your colon and fiber get to know each other better before jumping into a more serious relationship.

Vitamins and Minerals

Vitamins come from living sources such as animals and vegetables. Minerals come from inorganic, or dead, sources that were once part of a large rock or glacier, perhaps the earth's crust. Neither vitamins nor minerals will give you energy like fats, carbs, and proteins will, but that doesn't mean they're any less important. You need them for all of the chemical reactions in your body to occur. That may not seem like a very big deal, until you consider that those chemical reactions are responsible for everything from proper breathing to shiny hair.

You need over forty vitamins and minerals to keep your body humming along. Some of them, like vitamin C and calcium, you may be familiar with; others, like selenium and vanadium, you've probably never heard of. The point is, if you take in at least 1,600 calories a day (2,000 if you're a man, 38,000 if you're a water buffalo) in a diet consisting of 60 percent carbs, 20 percent proteins, and 20 percent fats, you should get a good percentage of the ones you need.

Of course, it's hard to strike the perfect balance of foods every day, especially if you're active or eat on the fly, so taking a vitamin and mineral supplement is a good idea as long as you don't expect magical results like a cure for baldness or a ten-point increase in your IQ from taking them. And don't get any ideas about vitamins taking the place of a good, healthy diet. A supplement is just a supplement, the way a Hamburger Helper without the Hamburger is just a Helper.

One more thing about vitamins: Don't be fooled by the slick marketing of expensive, designer supplements. Your body doesn't know the difference between a ten-dollar vitamin pill and a ten-cent vitamin pill. Most vitamins and minerals are water-soluble, so when your body uses the amount it needs, it dumps the rest rather than storing it. When you megadose on vitamins, chances are the only thing you're doing is producing very expensive urine. Don't be surprised if your urine turns strange shades of orange, gold, or green either. Supplements tend to do this.

However, certain vitamins, like A and D, are "fat-soluble"; in large doses the body treats them as toxic avengers. Rather than dumping excess amounts, your body stockpiles them until you're ready to use them. If you OD on supplements containing fat-soluble vitamins and don't use them quickly enough, they can have lethal effects.

Sodium

While it's a proven fact that eating a lot of sodium (salt) causes you to retain water—and appear as if you're retaining Häagen-Dazs—the research is a bit sketchy as to whether high sodium intake contributes to high blood pressure or any other type of physical malady. Nonetheless, we certainly eat more than we need; the average American eats between 5,000 and 7,000 milligrams of sodium daily when only about 2,500 milligrams (about a teaspoon) is truly required.

Your body easily replaces lost sodium, even if you sweat a lot. Traces of sodium are found naturally in virtually everything you eat. America pumps up the sodium content of raw foods in processing and packaging. According to Campbell's commercials, "soup is good food." And it is, for the most part, but unfortunately most soups contain over 1,000 milligrams of salt per serving. Limit your sodium intake by cutting back on canned food, prepared fast food, and highly packaged food. Or get versions of them that say "Low in Sodium" on the front. Keep in mind too that a typical fast-food meal delivers a quick 1,500 milligrams of salt. Usually a lot of fat too.

Water

Every single bodily function, from the simplest chemical reaction to the most complex movement, requires water. Water cools your body, aids circulation and digestion, and carries the fuel used to power your muscles. We need water as much as we need air. In fact, your body is about 60 percent water, and if you lose as little as 2 percent of your body weight through dehydration, your ability to think and move are seriously impaired.

Alcohol, caffeine, sun, heat, wind, exercise, smoking, and air conditioning are just a few of the things that can sap your body of water. You'll need to drink at least eight 8-ounce glasses of water to replenish what is lost through normal, everyday circumstances. You should drink two cups of water for every pound you lose from sweating. Obviously, you're not going to really know how much weight you've lost from sheer perspiration, but just be sure to drink a comfortable amount of water before and after exercising. And

glandular trivia The body has three million sweat glands. On a warm day during exercise the body will pump out 2 quarts of sweat. Thirsty?

171

then keep drinking a cup here or there whenever you get the chance. Your body can only absorb a small amount of liquid at a time, so replace lost water slowly, over the course of a few hours.

While it's important to drink several glasses of water a day, water can also come from other sources. Milk, for example, is nearly 90 percent water (try to stick to skim or low-fat milk). Juice, sports drinks, seltzer, even juicy fruits (that would be fruits that are juicy, not affiliated with the chewing gum of the same name)

count toward your daily water allotment. What doesn't count and even hurts, as we mentioned earlier, is alcohol and caffeinated drinks like coffee, tea (which has as much caffeine as coffee), and cola; all of these have a diuretic or dehydrating effect. Don't let 'em fool you just because they're liquids too; they'll quickly rob your body of water.

Caffeine

If you're one of those people who can't tie their shoes in the morning without a Java jolt, then you already know that caffeine is

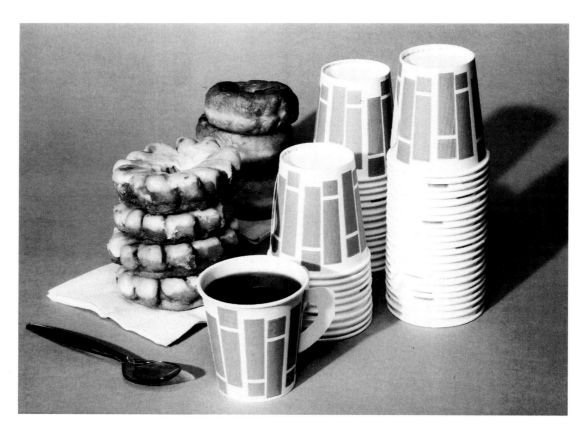

classified as a mild stimulant. It causes an increase in heart rate and metabolism which heightens mental sharpness for some. For others it causes behavior reminiscent of a cartoon cat, upside down, eyes bulging, and claws digging into the ceiling. Caffeine reaches the peak of its stimulating powers about thirty minutes after you've had that cup of coffee or tea. It takes your body four to six hours to metabolize half of your intake. By the way, it takes about ten hours for caffeine's effects to subside in women who use oral contraceptives. For smokers, about three hours.

Nutritional experts think that some caffeine won't hurt you but overindulging may have a negative impact on your health. Just what overdoing it means depends on your age, health, weight, and caffeine sensitivity, among other things. It seems most people are probably okay if they hold their caffeine intake to the equivalent of one to two cups of coffee (150 milligrams) a day.

So what is the downside to caffeine? In the short term, excessive caffeine consumption can result in mover-and-shaker syndrome: an agitated, nervous feeling, inability to concentrate, diarrhea, dehydration, and irritation. Caffeine can also inhibit your ability to absorb certain nutrients like thiamine, calcium, and iron. In the long term, heavy caffeine use has possible links to breast cancer, colon cancer, and osteoporosis, though the jury is still out.

On the flip side, caffeine has been used for thousands of years to gain a leg up on the competition in athletic events. Studies indicate that caffeine can increase endurance by enhancing fat utilization for energy and by dulling the pain of exercise so you don't feel like you're working as hard as you really are. There's a flip side to every flip side, however: beyond a cup and a half of coffee, caffeine has a diuretic effect and may bring on dehydration more quickly.

Bottom line? The pros and cons of caffeine are not written in stone. But it doesn't take an expert to tell you it's not good when your hands are shaking, you haven't slept in days, and you're crankier than Juan Valdés with a burro in heat.

Alcohol

In a way, alcohol is caffeine's opposite. It's a depressant that slows activity of the brain and spinal cord. But sometimes it's not such a bad idea to stop and smell the barley and hops. A cold beer after a run or a relaxing glass of wine with dinner are, for many of us, rituals worth rattling a few brain cells.

Don't sweat it if you like to knock back a few cold ones. It won't kill you, and

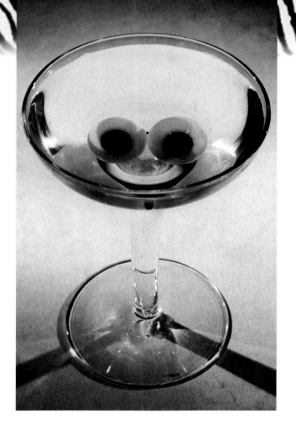

mixers like milk or cream) but your body prefers to metabolize these alcohol calories before it does anything else. So if you booze it up in combination with a fat-calorie laden meal, your body won't work on any of the fatty-food calories until it uses up the alcohol calories. Thus, a fattening meal becomes potentially even more fattening. Drinking adds pounds in other ways too, by increasing your appetite and decreasing your willpower. Everything looks better through beer goggles: strangers, co-workers, nachos, and, of course, another beer.

Obviously, you already know the dangers of overimbibing, but just in case you need to hear it again, heavy alcohol consumption damages every organ in your body, especially your heart. We're talking about heavy alcohol consumption, not a couple of drinks a day. For the average person, having more than six drinks a day on a regular basis damages the heart, puts extra stress on the damaged heart tissue, raises blood pressure, and leads to weight gain, which further stresses the heart. It destroys your liver and may contribute to the onset of osteoporosis. (It may take a little less if you're smaller than average, a little more if you're larger.) Last but not least, it impairs your good judgment and kills your motivation.

indeed there's evidence that it may increase your longevity by bolstering your immunity to heart disease and certain forms of cancer. By the way, you can get these benefits from any type of alcohol, not just red wine, as you may have heard. So, if a little alcohol is beneficial, then a lot must be really beneficial. Let's party! As logical as it *almost* sounds, it is unfortunately completely untrue.

You may want to skip that second beer for cosmetic reasons. Alcohol contributes toward weight gain. Not only does it deliver a whopping 7 calories per gram (mostly carb calories, very few fat calories unless you're adding fattening

Don't Put This in Your Mouth

It's easier to overdo your calorie intake and gain weight when your diet is high in fat. It's very simple. One gram of carbohydrate provides you with 4 calories of energy. Same for protein. But fat packs a 9-calorie punch per gram, so when you binge on a lot of junk food and fast food, you're getting double the amount of calories as when you eat the same amount of carbs or protein.

Even worse, fat calories are literally more fattening than other types of calories. About 23 percent of carb and protein calories are liberated through the heat of your body's chemical reactions—a process known as the thermal effect of food (TEF). Only about 3 percent of fat calories are lost through the thermal effect of food. The other 97 percent? If it isn't needed for fuel right away, it's stored as body fat. But remember, fat doesn't make people fat; people make people fat. As we've said, you do need a certain amount of fat to operate. Your goal should be to hover around that 20 percent range of daily fat intake.

Fat-Free Information

The proper way to cut out fat from your diet is to eat basic, simple foods as close to their natural state as possible: for ex-

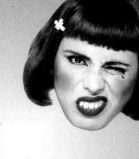

Julie's Nutrition Thoughts...

Diet Coke and Marlboro Lights is not eating light. You're smarter than that.

There's only one person who decides what goes in your mouth. And we know who that is.

ample, apples instead of apple pie, baked chicken instead of Kentucky Fried. As for those low-fat, no-fat, reduced-fat, fat-free cookies, cakes, pudding, breads, butter, and other fat-free stuff, here's a little fat-free information.

It's easy to be lulled into a false sense of security by products labeled "Fat-free!" Just be advised that fat-free doesn't mean scot-free. You may think it's okay to polish off a box of fat-free goodies, but you'll be getting hundreds more calories than you bargained for. Would you have eaten fewer of the better-tasting fat-filled kind? If you take in more calories than you burn, it doesn't matter if those calories come from carrots, lard, or fat-free ice cream. You're going to gain weight anyway.

There's another reason to reconsider fat-free treats: sugar. In an effort to pump up taste once the fat is removed, manufacturers often increase sugar (and sodium) content. Recent studies show that consuming too much sugar triggers your body's production of insulin, a hormone that encourages your body to hold on to body fat. Choose foods in which sugar is no higher than fourth on the list of ingredients; that includes synonymous substances such as honey, corn syrup, sucrose, and dextrose. And where there isn't sugar, there's NutraSweet, saccharine, or some other substitute sugar. Hey, they have to have some way to make this stuff taste good. And although they've been deemed safe by the FDA, we don't really know the long-term effects of these substances. We do know that some people get severe headaches from consuming massive quantities.

There's still another reason to limit your consumption of fat-free goodies. It's never been proven anywhere that these things help you lose weight. That goes for fat substitutes, diet sodas, and fake fats too. You have to watch how many calories you eat—not just how many "fat calories" you're consuming. If you eat high-calorie fat-free foods, you'll still be exceeding your body's calorie needs. And anyway, why not stick with naturally low-fat real foods with real nutrients that taste good?

Beware the New Nonfattening Fat

In a move that has enraged a number of nutrition experts, the FDA has given the okay to Olestra, the first fake fat to be approved for human consumption.

We already have tons of fat-free products on the market, so what's the big deal? Before Olestra came along, fat-free products were all made using fat substitutes derived from proteins and carbohydrates. They can't withstand high cooking temperatures, so they can't be used to make fried snack foods like chips and cheese puffs. So manufacturers have been left to use alternative processes such as baking, which is why most low-fat snack foods taste like plywood.

Olestra is different because it's bonafide *fat,* only it won't cost you 9 calories a gram. Olestra molecules are chemically designed to pass right through your body without being digested. An ounce of Olestra potato chips has little fat and just 70 calories, compared to 10 grams of fat and 150 calories in conventional chips.

So why are many health experts up in arms over the FDA's decision? Because when Olestra molecules pass through your body, they take certain nutrients right along with them. Some of these nutrients are thought to protect against cancer. Experts worry that people who consume massive quantities of Olestra products will be compromising their health. What's more, consuming moderate-to-large quantities of the stuff can cause severe diarrhea and abdominal discomfort in some people.

So here's a little advice: Don't look for Olestra (or the fat substitutes) to make all of your weight problems magically disappear. Go easy on processed snack foods. Instead, work on developing a taste for foods that are *naturally* low in fat.

A Good Plan for the Real World

Let's say you're at a cocktail party where the thought "If it's got a toothpick in it and I can eat it all in one bite, it doesn't really count" leads to (with the help of several plastic cups of Chardonnay) a whole box of toothpicks. Or, despite all of your willpower and better intentions you find your feet walking your mouth to that place where there's always plenty of fat in the fryer and never a cover charge—the Golden Arches. And then there are the holidays. That special time of year to get the family together and try once again to wipe out the entire turkey population.

These are the dilemmas of eating well on the cusp of the millennium. You may know everything there is to know on the subject, but in the end nutrition often comes down to pacing the aisles of a 7-Eleven, perusing the menu at the ballpark, or trying to decide if airport nachos are healthier than airport chili dogs.

While you wouldn't want to make a habit out of Happy Meals (or you won't be happy for long), an indulgence every once in a while is okay. Hey. We all gotta live, right? There are no wrong choices per se, just better choices to be made. Here's a look at some typical junk-food crisis situations and what the lesser evils are.

Fast Food

The best rule of thumb when having it your way is to keep it simple. Avoid specialty sandwiches with globs of special sauce and stick to pared-down, basic sandwiches or junior versions. Lose the words "cheese" and "double" from your order. If God had wanted us to have cheese with our burgers, he/she wouldn't have given us a way to get the milk out of the cow. Chicken and fish may seem like healthy alternatives, but if they're fried or batter-dipped, they rival specialty burgers in terms of fat and calories. That's true for anything that comes in chunk or nugget form as well. Many fast-food joints now

nutrition

"We are what we eat" is a function of "We are what we think." "I think I'll supersize my combo meal" leads to "I thought these jeans still fit me."

177

offer low-fat burger options, although the McDonald's McLean burger proved so unpopular it was dumped from the menu. A commentary on American eating habits or the fact that it tasted like wet clay? Better-tasting low-fat options include a barbecued chicken sandwich or a plain salad. Just go easy on the extras they put in "salads," like processed meats, cheese, and hard-boiled eggs and creamy dressings.

For McBreakfast, go with pancakes or an English muffin (hold the butter if you can stand it), orange juice, and low-fat milk. As for lunch, if you can, resist the 200-plus calories and 50 percent fat you'll get from a regular order of french fries. Go for the hot apple pie or chocolate shake instead. Though these two items offer nearly the same number of calories as the fries, more than half are from carbs and under 30 percent of their calories come from fat.

The best type of fast food can be found at pizza and Mexican chains. A slice of pizza is around 70 percent carbs and 20 percent fat (calories and fat vary by slice size, of course). Likewise for a bean burrito, an unadorned taco, or an order of rice and beans with a sprinkle of cheese.

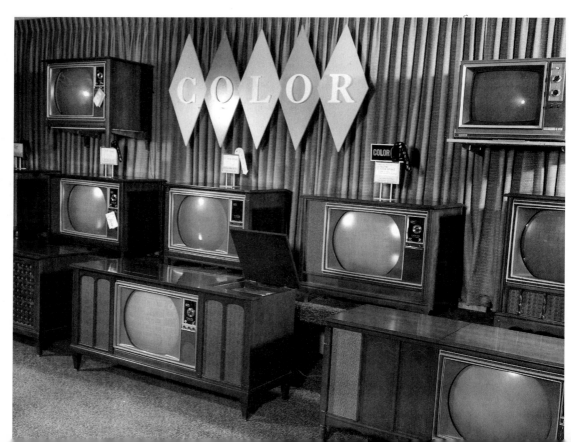

You do have to be careful, though. Taco Bell has one sandwich that weighs in at over 2,000 calories and 60 percent fat.

The Munchies

It's late at night, the flicker of the TV keeps you company like a loyal friend. Your eyes are busy, your mind is busy (sort of), your hands and your mouth are bored. A good time to recall that a measly 2-ounce bag of potato chips offers 306 calories, 58 percent of them from fat. Let's not even get into how much sodium they deliver. By comparison, a bag of tortilla chips has about the same number of calories but only half of them are from fat. (Still lots of salt, though.) That's better, but still not low enough. Nuts and seeds, though "natural," are even worse. They're small, they're cute, they're quiet, they're peanuts—they have something to hide. Ever looked at the back of the tiny airline package and gone into shock over the numbers? Yes, 320 calories for 2 ounces of peanuts and 77 percent of those calories are from fat.

Your best Crunch-y choice is a bag of pretzels, reduced salt if possible. Unlike chips and nuts, they're high in carbs, relatively low in calories, and only 6 percent fat. Tread carefully around popcorn. Air-popped without butter and salt offers just 20 low-fat calories per cup. But the same amount of microwave popcorn may deliver as many as 110 calories and 8 grams of fat.

In the creamy department, a cup of fruit-flavored, low-fat frozen yogurt is the safest selection (around 225 calories, 10 percent fat). But let the buyer beware: Frozen yogurt vendors are notoriously dishonest about fat, calorie, and sugar content and the serving sizes of their products. The most trustworthy are national brands you buy out of the carton. Even then, you should ignore the advertising weasel and read the nutritional labels carefully.

When you're in the mood for something sweet, and I bet you never thought a health book would be handing out this kind of advice, rip open a pack of Twinkies. Sure, they're pumped through with all kinds of chemicals, sugar, and God knows what else, but two of them are just 286 calories (68 percent from carbs and just 26 percent from fat) and now they have a lower-fat version. And you thought Twinkies couldn't get any lighter. Good to know when you've got a sweet tooth looking for the lesser of many evils.

Fig bars are your wisest cookie option (two have 110 calories, 17 percent fat). You can also try one of the low-fat cookie brands that seem to be breeding on super-

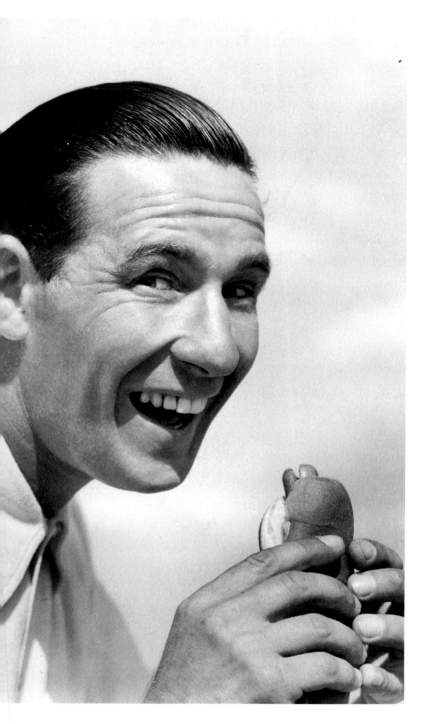

market shelves like rabbits. But do keep in mind that low fat does not guarantee low sugar or low calories. The same goes for low-fat cakes and pastries. It may ultimately be more satisfying and better to sample a few bites of the real McCoy.

The Ballpark

A professional sporting event is not the place to hang out when you're looking for a nutritious meal, but chances are you don't walk into the stadium every single night yelling "What's for dinner?" Probably the most damaging thing you can eat at the ballpark is the ballpark frank. They're essentially fat and nitrates on a bun, and to add insult to caloric injury, high hot-dog consumption has been identified as a risk factor for various types of cancer. So, want mustard with that?

Soft pretzels are probably the most benign sporting event snack; some parks now offer salt-free versions. If you've got a craving for peanuts, order them in the shell; they're still high in fat but hopefully the shells will slow you down so you'll have your fill before you get too carried away. And if you're lucky enough to live in a hip, happening, nutritionally aware kind of town, you'll find things like grilled chicken sandwiches, knishes, fruits, and salads at the concession stand. Otherwise, consider bringing your own packed lunch.

Travel

Unfortunately, many airlines still have jet lag as far as nutrition is concerned. We were served mystery meat topped with an unidentifiable sauce, a side of something swimming in butter, and a candy bar for dessert on a recent flight from New York to Dallas. Some have gotten their nutritional acts together, though; certain airlines now accommodate special food requests, often at no extra charge. Just call at least twenty-four hours in advance. Selections range from kosher to vegetarian and they're often of better quality than the usual thing because they are individually prepared.

Another airline pitfall: dehydration. Always drink plenty of water before, during, and after your flight. It's also best to stay away from alcohol and caffeinated drinks, which can further add to the dehydration effects of pressurized, recirculated air and altitude. Once you're earthbound again, you're often at the mercy of airport and hotel restaurants and you may have to search high and low for a piece of edible fruit or a main dish that isn't dripping with grease and fat. When good nutrition is hard to come by, that's the time vitamin supplements can come in handy, especially vitamin C, which helps counteract lowered resistance and close encounters with germs trapped in the plane's cabin.

Parties

The guests of honor at a party are often salty, fatty foods. They're pretty hard to resist, especially if you've had a little alcohol to lower your inhibition. Temptations notwithstanding, you can join the party without eating it.

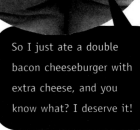

So I just ate a double bacon cheeseburger with extra cheese, and you know what? I deserve it!

Never go to a party hungry. You won't save calories by skipping a meal; in fact, if you haven't eaten for several hours, you're *more* likely to overeat. If possible, find out what's being served ahead of time, and if there aren't any low-fat options, be a gracious guest and bring your own. When you arrive, scan the buffet table and decide what you absolutely must try and what you can live without, keeping in mind everything you've just been taught. Grab a small plate and load it up with the must-try goodies. Eat slowly and wait at least twenty minutes before you go for refills. Make it a point to socialize with other people so you won't focus so much on eating. Have you ever noticed that people with the gift of gab always seem to be thinner? Science hasn't yet discovered whether thin people are annoyingly talkative or talkative people are annoyingly thin, although common sense seems to indicate that telling a really long story may help you keep from gaining weight.

As for alcohol, make sure you eat a little something before you start drinking so you won't drink too much too fast. Lower-calorie drinks include wine, wine spritzers, and light beer. If you find yourself guzzling, alternate alcoholic drinks with glasses of water or cut your wine or alcohol with generous amounts of juice, seltzer, or water. Decide on a maximum drink limit before the big party and then cut yourself off at that point. Eat something high in protein like a few pieces of low-fat cheese or a cup of yogurt to stave off a hangover. Some people even believe in taking a multiple vitamin with B complex. They say it helps in the morning. Which is good, because the morning is normally when you're quietly asking for help.

Party's Over

In spite of everything we told you, you went on a binge anyway. Well, relax. It's not like you're going to hell or anything, at least not for overeating. When you stray from your weight-loss program, what often hurts the most is not the extra calories you consume, but the way you react. You figure you blew it, so you keep right on eat-ing. There are more positive ways to counteract a lapse of control:

Stay Calm

The thing to do is to get back to normal as soon as possible. Even if you ate five pieces of cake the night before, don't skip breakfast the next morning. Starving yourself will just make matters worse and possibly send you into another binge spiral. Don't lose sight of the big picture: Think of a "slip" as getting temporarily off the track rather than permanent derailment.

Exercise

1,500 calories worth of cake and ice cream can be worked off by increasing your exercise session by 15 minutes a day for a week. Get a workout in as close to your binge as possible so fewer calories get a chance to lodge themselves in your body's fat stores. The extra exercise may also help dull your appetite and prevent the blowout from going any further.

Forgive Yourself

The important thing to remember is that nobody's perfect. Anxiety over a few extra cookies will only leave you ripe for another binge. What's done can't be undone, so the thing to do is to get on with your life and not worry so much about the past. You may want to give some thought as to why you lost it and then come up with a strategy to prevent future relapses.

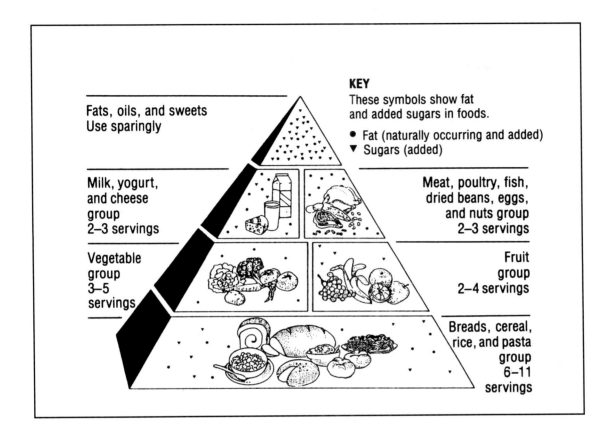

KEY
These symbols show fat and added sugars in foods.

- Fat (naturally occurring and added)
▼ Sugars (added)

Fats, oils, and sweets
Use sparingly

Milk, yogurt, and cheese group
2–3 servings

Meat, poultry, fish, dried beans, eggs, and nuts group
2–3 servings

Vegetable group
3–5 servings

Fruit group
2–4 servings

Breads, cereal, rice, and pasta group
6–11 servings

Getting Over the Hangover

Your pants are off, your boots are still on. You wonder how. You also wonder where that fifty-franc note and old paperback copy of *Breakfast at Tiffany's* came from. The alcohol is doing a victory lap around your brain, banging pots, pans, and cymbals. How do you get rid of it? Unfortunately, the only cure for a hangover is time. Your body metabolizes about one-third of an ounce of alcohol per hour: a little less than the amount in a 12-ounce beer, a 5-ounce glass of wine, or the average mixed drink. Drinking coffee to snap out of it will only make you a more alert drunk.

In the meantime, a few things can help ease your suffering. Get as much rest as you can and avoid bright lights if possible. Take an aspirin or aspirin substitute to help ease the overall ache. Drink as much water as your stomach can handle. Juice isn't such a good idea because the acid may further upset your stomach.

Excess, no good. Moderation, good. You've heard it before. Live modestly. Enjoy the good stuff in moderation. It seems so ridiculously obvious, yet the temptation to overdo on all the good stuff seems to get the best of all of us. That, and the temptation to sit on our asses tend to take over once we've overdone all the good stuff.

The Food Pyramid

In 1992, the federal government exiled the Four Food Groups and unveiled the Food Guide Pyramid. Although the new plan looks like a complete departure from the four basics, it's simply a more detailed look at the same picture.

The lion's share of your calories should come from the foods at the bottom of the pyramid: grains, cereals, rice, pasta, fruits, and vegetables. Meat, poultry, fish, eggs, and dairy products fall in the center, and fats, oils, and sweets are at the very top, under the heading of "use sparingly." The pyramid isn't perfect; for instance, it doesn't distinguish between saturated fats (found in meat and dairy products) and the healthier unsaturated fats. To make sure you don't go overboard on calories, pay attention to what counts as a "serving." For instance, according to the pyramid, a "serving" of pasta is a half cup. The federal government's idea of a meat serving, 3 ounces, is about the size of a deck of cards. Here's a rundown of serving sizes as defined by the government:

Fats, oils, sweets: Use sparingly. This means as little as possible—or, according to most health organizations, less than 30 percent of your total calories. *Meat, poultry, fish, dry beans, eggs, nuts:* One serving equals 2–3 ounces of lean cooked meat, fish, or poultry; 1 egg; ½ cup of cooked beans; 2 tablespoons of seeds and nuts. *Milk, yogurt, cheese:* One serving equals one cup of milk or yogurt, enough to fill your cereal bowl in the morning; or about a slice and a half of pre-cut cheese. Choose the low-fat varieties. *Fruits:* One serving equals one medium apple, banana, or orange; ½ cup of chopped fruit or berries; ¾ cup of fruit juice. Fresh fruits are preferable to frozen, canned, dried, or juiced. *Vegetables:* One serving equals 1 cup of raw leafy vegetables; ½ cup of other vegetables chopped; ¾ cup of vegetable juice. *Bread, cereal, rice, pasta:* One serving equals 1 slice of bread; 1 ounce of ready-to-eat cereal; ½ cup of cooked cereal, rice, or pasta.

Vitamin	RDA	Function	Good Sources
Thiamin (B1)	1.5 mg	Without it, you won't burn carbohydrates. It also plays a special role in keeping your heart, nerves, and brain functioning properly.	Lean meat, pasta, organ meats, green peas, legumes, oranges, asparagus, whole grains
Riboflavin (B2)	1.7 mg	Lack of B2 can lead to dry, scaly skin plus you'll have trouble seeing in bright light.	Organ meats, dairy, oysters, lean meats, chicken, dark green leafy vegetables, sardines, eggs, tuna, whole grains, legumes
Niacin (B3)	20 mg	Keeps LDL cholesterol under control and plays a role in processing carbs. Don't megadose on it, though. This can lead to liver damage.	Lean meats, fish, poultry, nuts, legumes, dark green leafy vegetables, whole grains, eggs
Pyridoxine (B6)	2 mg	Helps break down proteins and is an ingredient in some essential amino acids. Helps pump up your immune system too.	Lean meat, liver, fish, nuts, legumes, whole grains, poultry, corn, bananas
Cyanocobalamin (B12)	6 micrograms	Lack of B12 can lead to anemia (not enough red blood cells). Kids need it for strong bones and muscles.	Organ meats, lean meat, egg yolks, dairy, fish, shellfish
Folic Acid	400 micrograms	It may lower some birth defects and some experts now think it may lower the risk of heart disease and some cancers.	Meat, dark green leafy vegetables, asparagus, lima beans, whole grains, nuts, legumes
Ascorbic Acid (C)	60 mg	No proof yet that C helps prevent colds but it still may help boost immunity. It helps build healthy bones, teeth, and skin. Smokers use up C more rapidly, so should get an extra dose of it.	Strawberries, citrus fruit, cauliflower, cabbage, tomatoes, asparagus

Vitamin	RDA	Function	Good Sources
A	1,000 retinal equivalents	Eat plenty of vitamin A for healthy skin and sharp eyesight.	Liver, eggs, dairy, dark green leafy vegetables, apricots, peaches, cantaloupes, carrots, squash
D	400 international units	Builds strong bones. Helps the body absorb and use calcium.	Milk, egg yolks, fortified breakfast cereals, sunlight
E	30 international units	Lack of E leads to anemia and dull, lifeless skin and hair.	Plant oils, wheat germ, dark green leafy vegetables, nuts, whole grains, liver, egg yolks, legumes, most other fruits and vegetables
K	80 micrograms	Helps stave off bone density loss and also helps wounds to heal. Essential for normal kidney functioning.	Dark green leafy vegetables, asparagus, spinach, turnip greens

Mineral	RDA	Purpose	Source
Calcium	1,200 mg	Keeps your bones strong now and in the future. Also helps keep your blood pressure low and possibly wards off colon cancer.	Dairy, dark green leafy vegetables, broccoli, fortified orange juice
Chromium	none	Regulates blood sugar.	Brewer's yeast, meat, clams, whole grains, cheeses, nuts
Copper	2 mg	Bolsters the immune system. Too little of it may contribute to high total cholesterol levels.	Organ meats, shellfish, whole grains, nuts, legumes, lean meat, fish, fruits, vegetables
Iodine	150 micrograms	Helps regulate metabolism.	Iodized salt, seafood, seaweed, dairy, meats
Iron	18 mg	Without it, expect a lack of energy due to anemia. (Women in particular are prone to iron deficiencies.)	Organ meats, red meat, fish, shellfish, poultry, enriched cereals, egg yolks, dark green leafy vegetables, dried fruits
Magnesium	400 mg	Fundamental for numerous functions. Adequate magnesium intake may prevent the formation of kidney stones.	Whole grains, nuts, legumes, dark green leafy vegetables, seafood, chocolate
Phosphorus	1,000 mg	Essential for strong bones and teeth and healthy skin. Most Americans get too much of it from soft drinks and processed foods.	Dairy, fish, meat, poultry, egg yolks, nuts, legumes, whole grains, soft drinks, processed foods
Potassium	none	Regulates the body's fluid balance. Helps keep blood pressure low.	Lean meat, fresh fruits and vegetables, dairy, nuts, legumes
Selenium	none	Helps the heart and immune system function properly. May help prevent some forms of cancer.	Organ meats, seafood, lean meats, whole grains, dairy
Zinc	15 mg	Men, you need zinc for proper sperm production. Women, zinc helps normal development of the fetus. It helps heal wounds and boost immunity no matter what sex you are.	Meat, poultry, eggs, oysters, dairy, whole grains

MINERALS

Source	Serving Size	Grams of Fiber
Apple	1, medium	3
Broccoli	½ cup, fresh	2.5
Brown Rice	½ cup, cooked	1.7
Carrots	½ cup, fresh	2.5
Corn	½ cup, niblets	3
Corn Bran	2 Tbsp., raw	8
Farina	¾ cup, cooked	2.5
Figs	2, medium	4
Kidney Beans	1 cup, cooked	10
Lentils	1 cup, cooked	8
Lima Beans	½ cup, boiled	6.6
Oatmeal	¾ cup, cooked	4
Orange	1, medium	4
Popcorn	3 ½ cups, popped	4.5
Prunes	5, medium	3
Raisins	½ cup	4
Spaghetti	1 cup, cooked	2.2
Spinach	1 cup, fresh, chopped	4
Squash	1 cup, cooked	6
Strawberries	1 cup, fresh	4

Food	Calories	% Fat	Sodium (mg)	Cholesterol (mg)
Chicken				
Burger King Chicken Sandwich	685	40	1,417	65
Kentucky Fried Chicken—Light N' Crispy Drumstick	121	52	196	61
Extra Crispy Thigh	406	67	688	129
McDonald's Chicken McNuggets	270	50	580	56
Wendy's Chicken Club Sandwich	506	44	930	70
Hamburgers				
Burger King	272	36	505	37
McDonald's	260	35	500	37
Roy Rogers	456	55	495	73
Wendy's	260	31	570	34
Specialty Sandwiches				
Burger King Whopper	626	55	842	94
McDonald's Big Mac	570	55	979	83
McDonald's Quarter Pounder w/cheese	525	54	1220	107
Wendy's Big Classic	570	52	1085	90
French Fries				
Burger King, regular	227	52	160	14
McDonald's, regular	220	47	109	9
Roy Rogers, regular	268	45	165	42
Wendy's, regular	280	45	95	15

huh?

A Glossary of Terms in Case You Forget

Aerobic: Sustained exercise, such as walking, running, or cycling, which requires oxygen for fuel. Involves the repetitive, rhythmic movement of large muscle groups, such as your buns and thighs, and causes an elevation in heart rate. The most efficient calorie and fat-burning form of exercise.

Aerobic Heart Rate Zone: 70–80 percent of maximum heart rate. A challenging but doable pace. For more advanced exercisers doing up to 30 minutes of cardiovascular training. Increases your stamina and strength.

Alignment: Also referred to as posture. Natural alignment is an ideal posture in which your head is centered between your shoulders, your shoulders are relaxed backward and downward, your chest and rib cage are lifted, your abdominals are pulled in toward your spine, your lower body is relaxed, and your weight is distributed evenly between both feet.

Anaerobic: Short bursts of exercise, usually lasting less than a minute, designed to increase the power, strength, and tone of a muscle. It relies on cellular enzymes rather than oxygen for fuel. Example: target toning.

Anaerobic Threshold Heart Rate Zone: 80–90 percent of maximum heart rate. Several 2–10 minute intervals at this level done once or twice a week will help advanced exercisers develop speed and power.

Awareness Exercise: Awareness exercises teach you how your abs and lower-back muscles relate to the rest of your body. Also work the transversus abdominus, a muscle group that only contracts when you pull your abs in toward your spine and exhale.

Basal Metabolic Rate (BMR): Number of calories you need per day for basic bodily functions. For most women this number is around 1,000 calories; for men, around 1,400.

Body-Fat Percentage: A method of determining how much of your weight is fat and how much is lean body tissue (muscle). Optimal body-fat percentage for women is 16–26 percent; for men, 12–20 percent.

Body Weight: Your weight in pounds. Usually taken on a scale. This measure does not distinguish how much of your body composition is fat and how much is muscle.

Calorie: Unit to measure energy from food.

Cardiovascular: Exercise that works the heart and lungs and, if done on a regular basis, increases endurance and the efficiency of oxygen usage.

Contraction: When a muscle responds to a force by shortening, lengthening, or pushing against it without changing length. A contraction is experienced in the form of tension in the muscle being worked.

Cool-down: A period immediately following exercise during which light activities, such as slow walking and stretching, are done in order to gradually slow your heart rate, breathing, and general metabolism.

Ectomorph: A body type characterized by hips and shoulders approximately the same width, small-to-medium bones, and a lanky, angular appearance.

Endomorph: A body type characterized by hips wider than the shoulders, large bones, and a curvy, rounded appearance.

Ergonomics: Setting up your work environment for maximum efficiency and comfort.

Exercise: Refers to the actual movement you are doing in a workout. For instance a Squat in a buns workout or a Wall Sit in a leg workout.

Exercise Light: Theory which states you need only accumulate 30 minutes or more of moderately intense activity most—preferably all—days of the week to produce an aerobic training effect. Under this definition, pastimes as informal as gardening and house painting are considered exercise.

Extension Exercise (Abdominals): Exercises which result in a lengthening of the spine. Work the erector spinae muscles of the lower back.

Fat-Burning Zone: Bogus theory which states that long, slow, low-intensity aerobic work is the best way to lose body fat because more fat is used as fuel at lower exercise intensities.

Fitness: The ability to function optimally. Fitness level refers to your present level of physical condition.

Flexibility: Refers to the degree of mobility or the range of motion a joint can move through. A consistent program of stretching exercises increases flexibility.

Forward Flexion Exercise (Abdominals): Bending forward at the waist. Better known as the traditional Crunch. These exercises strengthen the rectus abdominus, the long, thin, flat muscle which runs from just below your breastbone and attaches to your pelvis.

Functional Flexibility: The minimum amount of joint flexibility to perform ordinary tasks.

Heart Rate: The number of times your heart beats per minute. Usually measured by taking your pulse by palpating your radial artery for fifteen seconds and then multiplying the number of beats counted by 4.

Intensity: The quality of effort you put into a workout or individual exercise.

Kyphosis: Excessively rounded or droopy shoulders. Common cause of neck and back pain.

Locked: Refers to a joint such as the knee or elbow when it is fully extended or "hyperextended." This puts undo pressure on the joint and throws off body alignment.

Lordosis: Excessively arched back. Common source of lower-back discomfort.

Lower Flexion (Abdominals): Reverse Crunches or any movements that involve lifting your hips upward while your upper body remains anchored. Work the entire rectus with special emphasis on the lower half.

Macronutrient: Carbohydrates, proteins, and fats. Broken down by the body for fuel.

Maximum Heart Rate: The maximum number of times your heart is capable of beating per minute. Declines about one beat each year; estimated by the age-predicted method (subtracting your age from 220).

Mesomorph: A body type characterized by shoulders slightly wider than the hips, medium-to-large bones, and a muscular, athletic appearance.

Micronutrient: Vitamins and minerals. Need only small amounts for usage in bodily functions.

Mind/Body Focus: Something that helps link your thought process with your body's movement—that is, thinking with your muscles. Often this is done by relating the movement to something that is familiar.

Moderate Heart Rate Zone: 50–60 percent of maximum heart rate. For workouts lasting longer than 60 minutes or for beginning aerobicizers.

Periodization: When you cycle the difficulty and amount of training you do over an extended period of time. Variables which can be modified include sets, reps, weights, number of exercises, and amount of rest between exercises. Usually refers to resistance training but can be applied to any type of

Cardiovascular, also known as cardio. Do cardio enough and it'll keep you from gasping for air while you're doing cardio.

Your target-training zone . . . you can get there from here.

Intensity: a quality workout requires focus and concentration. When you go to the gym it's best to bring your mind along as well.

training. There are five periodization phases: Prep, Pump, Peak, Push, and Rest.

Radial Artery: A point on the side of your wrist directly below your thumb where your pulse is located.

Rating of Perceived Exertion (RPE): A method of measuring intensity which utilizes a scale to relate your perception of the difficulty to the physical effort of the exercise.

Red-Line Heart Rate Zone: 90–100 percent of maximum heart rate. Used for exercise intervals lasting no more than 60 seconds and only if you are extremely fit and peaking for a competition.

Repetition: A complete movement of an exercise. Also: rep. Plural: reps.

Resistance Training: Also known as strength or weight training. When you work your muscles against a load or resistance. Commonly used forms of resistance are body weight, dumbbells, weight machines, and exercise bands.

Rest: The briefest possible interval between sets which allows the working muscle to regain full strength. Also: the time interval between workouts.

Rotation Exercise (Abdominals): Any exercise that involves twisting from the middle or bending to the side. Works the internal and external obliques, the muscles that attach to the sides of your torso.

Routine: A group of exercises.

Set: A group of continuously performed repetitions. In target toning, a set consists of 8–15 repetitions.

Soft: Not fully straightened, as it applies to a joint such as the knee or elbow.

Split Routine: A method of training in which different muscle groups are target-toned on different days.

Spot Reducing: An ineffective method of training which involves performing a high number of repetitions at a low intensity.

Stabilization Exercise (Abdominals): Exercise in which your abdominal and lower-back muscles contract to keep your spine upright and stabilized.

Steady-State Heart Rate Zone: 60–70 percent of maximum heart rate. For workouts lasting 30–60 minutes. Beginners who are ready to push a little harder can crisscross intervals at this pace with Moderate Heart Rate Zone intervals.

Super Circuit: A method of training in which a brief interval of an aerobic activity is alternated with a set of target toning with no rest period in between.

Super Set: A technique that involves combining two sets of two different exercises with no rest in between.

Talk Test: A method of determining aerobic exercise intensity in which you gauge the difficulty of talking as you exercise.

Target Heart Rate Range: The number of times your heart beats per minute in the range that keeps you aerobically exercising at the appropriate intensity level. The most common method of determining this is with the age-predicted formula: subtract your age from 220 and then multiply it by 60 and 85 percent (e.g., 0.60 and 0.85).

Thermal Effect of Food (TEF): Calories liberated through the heat of your body's chemical reactions.

Training Range: The minimum and the maximum workout intensity for safe and effective exercise. Usually measured by heart rate.

Warm-up: The period of time when you engage in light activities such as walking or easy jogging in order to prepare your body for hard physical exercise. The warm-up period increases the blood flow to your muscles, speeds up heart rate, and elevates body temperature.

end!

Let's just have a quick sum-up of what we've learned about fitness.

Get 20 minutes of aerobic exercise at least three times a week. More if you want to lose weight; see the "Move!" chapter and review it if you don't remember.

Strength-train three or four times a week, allowing your muscles 24 hours to rest between workouts; see the "Pump!" chapter and review. You'll probably be referring back to this chapter the most since you'll need to reread the exercise instructions for a while to get the routine down.

Keep a record of your "inches lost," "fat lost," "strength gained" as you undertake our fitness program and watch how your natural body shape and fitness level begins to change and improve. See the "Flesh!" chapter for a review and for the comparison box you'll need to record improvements.

Stretch after your workouts. Flexibility is part of being fit. It helps your muscles feel better, react to exercise better, and may even protect you against injury. See the "Stretch!" chapter for a review and to relearn the exercises so you can easily fit them in after your strength-training routine.

Try to eat a nutritionally balanced diet consisting of 60 percent carbohydrate, 20 percent protein, and 20 percent fat. How you eat will greatly influence your fitness level and aid you in weight control. Don't crash-diet. Losing a lot of weight suddenly can lower your metabolism and make you gain more weight later. And if you have to overdo it on the bad stuff every so often, go ahead. This may help you keep to a healthier diet in the long run. Review the "Chow!" chapter every so often to help yourself remember the guidelines.

Do all of this stuff. Get it? This is the Crunch Fitness Program and it's pretty simple. We didn't say easy, just simple. Hopefully, we're not asking too much. Most of it is just good common sense and works well into just about everyone's lifestyle. We just want you to be good to yourself. Believe in yourself and it will happen. Get a taste of exercise and you'll probably keep doing it. You owe it to yourself. Maybe it will lead to other great and challenging things as you become fitter, stronger, more confident, calm, and happy. Good luck. And remember, if you're ever in New York or LA, stop into Crunch and show off your Crunch Book improvements for us. Maybe stay long enough for a gospel aerobics class. It's not a must. Remember: At Crunch, everyone is welcome and fitness is fun. We hope it will be for you.

About the author, and other folks who sacrificed their fitness for the sake of this book:

Liz Neporent, who holds a master's degree in exercise physiology and fitness management, is president of Frontline Fitness and a renowned fitness consultant and writer. Liz is the co-author of *Buns of Steel: The Total Body Workout, Abs of Steel,* and *Fitness for Dummies.* She's the fitness editor for *Women's Sports and Fitness Magazine* and writes regularly for magazines such as *Shape, Men's Fitness,* and *Family Circle.* An expert on health and fitness, Liz appears regularly on CBS, Fox's *Noon News,* CNBC, the TV Food Network, and various other TV and radio programs. She is certified by the American College of Sports Medicine, the American Council on Exercise, the National Strength and Conditioning Association, and the National Academy of Sports Medicine.

John Egan is an advertising copywriter who broke every rule in this book while working on it. John is currently still trying to weasel a free membership in Crunch in New York City.

Sarah Dent, creative director at Crunch, produced this book. Sarah's responsibilities included organizing the photo shoots, selecting images, editing the text, and wearing a chicken suit.